P.LATES
for pregnancy

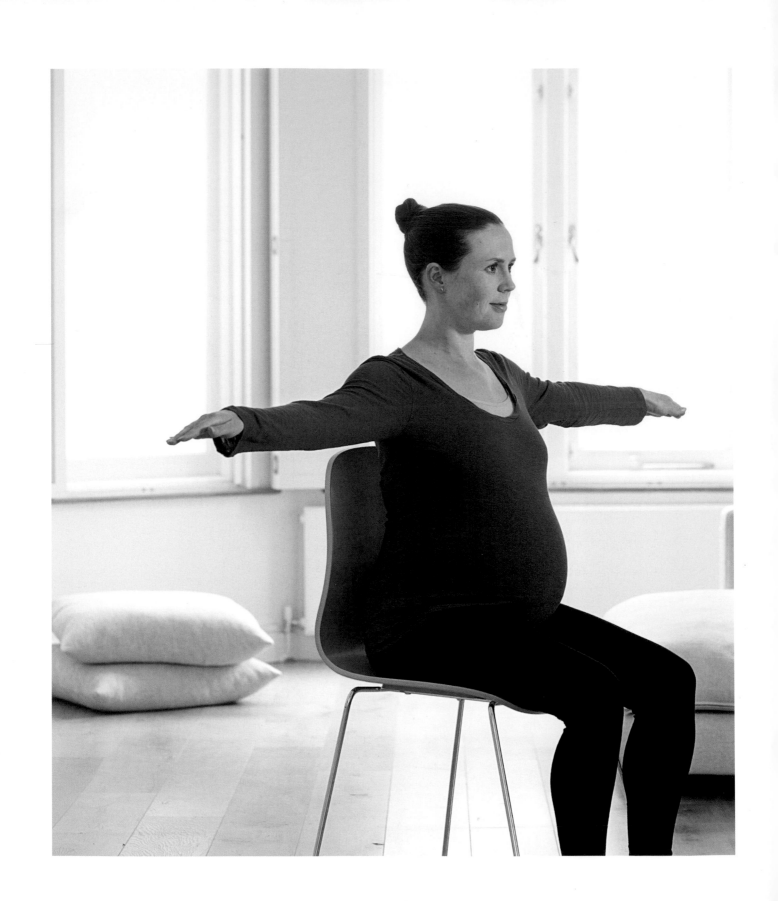

PILATES
for pregnancy

The ultimate exercise guide to see you through pregnancy and beyond

Lynne Robinson

with Kate Fernyhough MCSP

PHOTOGRAPHY BY DAN DUCHARS

Kyle Books

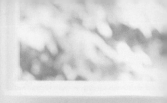

First published in Great Britain in 2012 by
Kyle Books
23 Howland Street, London W1T 4AY
general.enquiries@kylebooks.com
www.kylebooks.com
10 9 8 7 6 5 4 3 2 1
ISBN 978-0-85783-052-4

Disclaimer The author and publisher cannot accept any
responsibility for misadventure resulting from the practice
of any of the techniques or principles in this book. It is not
intended to be and should not be used as guidance for the
treatment of serious healthy problems; please refer to a medical
professional if you have concerns about any aspect of your
condition or fitness level.

Lynne Robinson is hereby identified as the author of this work
in accordance with Section 77 of the Copyright, Designs and
Patents Act 1988.

Text © 2011 Lynne Robinson
Book design © 2011 Kyle Books
Photographs © 2011 Dan Duchars

Project editor: Jenny Wheatley
Photographer: Dan Duchars
Designer: Jane Humphrey
Illustrator: John Erwood
Hair and Make-up: Marie Anne Coulter using Bobbie Brown
Proofreader: Elizabeth Rees Evans
Models: Joy Broadway, Sally Brown, Sally Buliga, Elena
Carofyllakis, Steph Davies, Lina Granborg, Anaya Grover,
Kate Hodder, Claire Lydon-Strutt, Eilis Macleod, Karen Shaw,
Lindsay Taylor, Matteo Warden, Sarah-Louise Warden
Production: Nic Jones and David Hearn

A Cataloguing In Publication record for this title is
available from the British Library.

Colour reproduction by Alta Image, London.
Printed and bound by Toppan Leefung Printing Ltd.

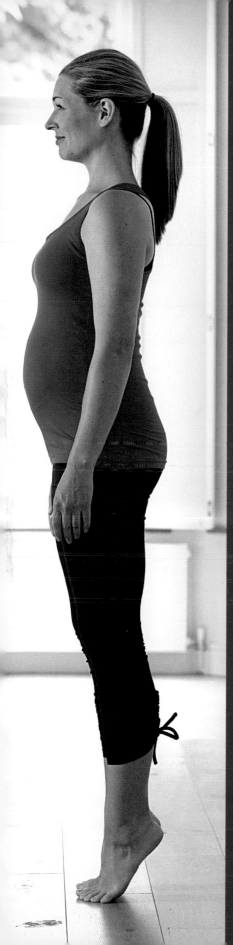

contents

Foreword   7

Introduction   8

What are the benefits of this Pilates programme?   9

About this book   10

How to use the antenatal programme   11

Your changing body (and how Pilates can help)   12

Before you begin   28

Learning the Fundamentals of Pilates   30

Preparing for Pregnancy   74

The Early Pregnancy Programme   110

The Later Pregnancy Programme   132

Preparing for Labour and the Birth   168

After the Birth   188

Index   220

Further information   223

Acknowledgements   224

Foreword

This book, written by the world's bestselling Pilates author Lynne Robinson, and supported by physiotherapy and midwifery advisors, is a clearly written and generously illustrated one-stop resource for any stage of pregnancy. It describes the stages and changes that occur during pregnancy and demonstrates safe Pilates exercises, with modifications where necessary, that can be adapted to the pregnant woman and her evolving shape. It discusses the contraindications to exercise in pregnancy, and gives helpful advice and exercises for common problems encountered during pregnancy such as incontinence and diastasis recti. It also describes ways in which to prepare for the birth, including how to relax the pelvic floor as well as breathing techniques to assist relaxation during pregnancy and the inevitable tricky stages of labour. The book then offers programmes for women who have had a normal vaginal delivery, assisted delivery and caesarean births, helping to restore normal function.

There is emerging evidence that pelvic floor muscle (PFM) training before, during and after pregnancy can reduce the incidence of pelvic floor disorders such as incontinence, prolapse and pelvic pain. PMF training during pregnancy has also been shown to lower the rate of prolonged second stage of labour. If that was not enough, since back pain during pregnancy is linked to increased odds of developing a pelvic floor disorder, maintaining good postural awareness and muscle function during pregnancy seems very sensible to say the least! Physical activity is safe for most pregnant women and improves maternal fitness and birth outcomes, furthermore it is reported that regular physical activity not only improves self-esteem, it can reduce symptoms of anxiety and depression during pregnancy.

So if you're pregnant, hoping to become pregnant, already a new mum, new to Pilates or a veteran – even if you don't think you have the time to read, never mind actually exercise – I wholeheartedly recommend this book, which will be a welcome addition to your home for years to come.

Dr Ruth Lovegrove Jones PhD MCSP

Ruth combines the disciplines of international research, writing and education alongside her role as a clinician. She has worked in private practice for the last 20 years, establishing a multidisciplinary clinic for pain management, sports medicine and pelvic floor rehabilitation.

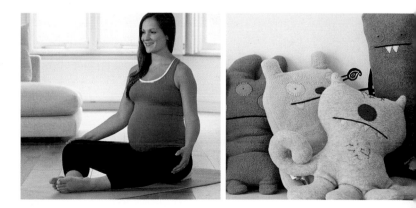

Introduction

So you are going to have a baby? Or perhaps you are planning on having a baby?

As any mother will tell you, no two babies are the same. No two pregnancies. No two labours or deliveries. While we can, and will, give you an outline of what to expect during your pregnancy and labour, no one can be sure what exactly will happen. However, there is one thing we can be sure about. The better prepared you are, the fitter and healthier you are, the better chance you and your baby have of being healthy.

While motherhood is undeniably the most exciting and rewarding journey any woman can take, it has its challenges. Pregnancy is a natural condition, you are part of the cycle of life yet you will be physically, mentally and emotionally stretched. Your body will become softer and more flexible due to hormonal changes. Every one of your body's systems will be affected. There may be times when, in spite of the joy of carrying a new life, your body does not feel like your own.

The exercises in this book are specially designed to help you cope with these changes. The programme can help you learn how to use your body well and have confidence in your ability to manage your pregnancy, your labour and the birth itself.

The sooner you start the better. If you are thinking of starting a family, or expanding your existing one, you will want to adopt a healthy lifestyle now. Sweep out the cobwebs. This will involve eating a healthy balanced diet, exercising and getting plenty of rest and relaxation. Then, once you are pregnant, exercising will already be part of your regular routine. Staying active throughout your pregnancy is key. You are going to need to be fit to deliver, as labour is what the name suggests – hard work!

As a pregnant woman your exercise needs will change as your pregnancy progresses. We will be looking at the ways in which your body is adapting, and the impact this has on how you should exercise. With this in mind, after the chapter on Preparing for Pregnancy, we have divided the programme into Early Pregnancy and Later Pregnancy. There is a special chapter on Preparing for Labour and the Birth and one devoted to After the Birth. There is even a section on how to work out with your baby!

Taking into account the latest medical advice on contraindicated movements and positions, you can be assured that Body Control Pilates is the safest, most effective and, hopefully, the most enjoyable exercise method that you can do at this very exciting time.

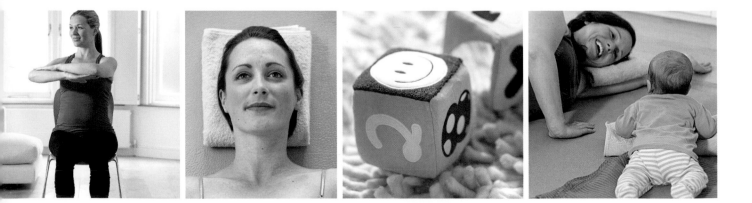

What are the Benefits of this Pilates Programme?

Pilates is a complete mind and body training method. But if you wanted to describe it simply, it is mindful movement. The exercises within this book are based on Body Control Pilates, a school of Pilates renowned for its safe but effective approach. It only takes one glance at the Eight Principles which underlie Body Control Pilates to appreciate just how suitable it is for pregnancy:

Concentration	Centring
Relaxation	Co-ordination
Alignment	Flowing Movements
Breathing	Stamina

These are all skills you are going to need during your pregnancy, labour and for motherhood itself!

So why choose Pilates for your pre-pregnancy, ante- and postnatal exercise regime?

Pre-pregnancy

x To help prepare you and your body before you become pregnant. The gentle exercises, together with healthy lifestyle changes, can help you achieve a healthy pre-pregnancy weight. This is important as research has shown that being over- or underweight is detrimental to becoming pregnant as well as to your baby's health.

* To help you relax, de-stress and feel more positive about yourself.

Antenatal

* To improve your body awareness so that you are in tune with your body and growing baby.

* To help with the changes to your posture caused by your overall weight gain and the additional weight of the growing baby, uterus and breasts.

* To help with the hormonal changes and the effect of ligamentous laxity on your joints.

* To develop your natural 'corset' to support your back and baby.

* To prepare your body for the carrying of the baby.

* For the health of all your body's systems: circulatory; lymphatic; respiratory; digestive and reproductive.

* For breathing and relaxation skills, so important throughout your pregnancy and for the labour itself.

* To help you to understand and stay in harmony with your body, to learn to work with it through labour, not against it. Many of the exercises may encourage the baby to be in the right presentation. There are also exercises to help you be comfortable in many common birthing positions.

* For pelvic floor education and control, including how to release your pelvic floor for the baby's delivery.

And for after the birth

* To get you ready for all the demands of motherhood – a lot of bending, kneeling and carrying.

* To help you regain abdominal tone and improve the abdominal divide (diastasis recti) if present.

* During pregnancy your ribcage lifts and flares to accommodate the growing baby, Pilates can help encourage the ribs to close back down.

* To restore the pelvic floor, helping with pelvic floor problems such as stress incontinence.

* To help prevent common joint problems, including pelvic girdle pain.

* To release endorphins, the 'feel-good' hormones.

* For your mental health, helping you to de-stress and learn how to relax.

* Last, but by no means least, to help you manage your weight, tone up and get back into shape!

About this Book

One of our main goals in putting this Pilates programme together was to choose exercises that will help you to understand and become aware of your body and its needs. Unless you have been pregnant before, everything is going to feel strange and new. Understanding the changes your body is going through is as important to your self-awareness and body confidence as the exercises themselves. So take time to read through 'Your changing body' before you begin. This section will give you valuable insight not only into the changes but why and how Pilates is so beneficial, and why you will need to modify your Pilates practice along the way.

The Preparing for Pregnancy chapter is perfect if you are planning a natural conception. The exercises are also suitable if you are planning fertility treatment although you will need to check with your medical consultant. Your partner will also want to be in good health so perhaps they could join in too. Be sure to work through The Fundamentals first.

Once you think you may be pregnant, stop and seek further medical advice before continuing onto the antenatal exercises. We cannot stress enough the importance of medical permission to start the programme even if you believe you have a normal pregnancy.

Only your medical practitioner will know your detailed medical history. Then ask again at regular intervals, perhaps at your antenatal clinic visits as your ability to exercise may change.

The exercises themselves are divided into Early and Later Pregnancy. The reason we have divided them in this way is that we recommend that mothers-to-be who are new to Pilates wait until 16 weeks before joining the programme. Trying to start a new exercise regime when you are also trying to cope with all the changes of pregnancy may prove too much of a challenge. But by 16 weeks the placenta is fully formed, your pregnancy is well under way and you should be more comfortable with your body. Sixteen weeks also happens to be a perfect time to modify some of the positions and movements in the programme.

So, to recap, if you have never done Pilates before, or perhaps have only tried a few sessions, we would recommend that you wait until you are at least 16 weeks pregnant before starting the programme (if in doubt, simply follow the flowchart opposite).

Then, after reading through the opening chapters, turn to page 150 where you will be shown which exercises to choose from The Fundamentals for Later Pregnancy. After mastering these Fundamentals you can then join The Later Pregnancy programme.

On the other hand, if you have been doing regular Pilates for at least 4–6 months, with your doctor's clearance, you may revise The Fundamentals and then start the Early Pregnancy Programme, progressing to The Later Pregnancy Programme at about 16 weeks.

If you have picked up this book after the birth of your baby, you will need medical clearance to start exercising and then, once again, you will need to learn The Fundamentals before starting the postnatal exercises.

If you have been with us throughout your pregnancy, well done! You should be able to start the postnatal programme as soon as your doctor or midwife gives you the all-clear, which for normal deliveries is usually around 6 weeks postnatal.

How to Use the Antenatal Programme

The antenatal programme is divided into two sections, for Early and Later Pregnancy. This is because as a pregnancy progresses past 16 weeks, certain positions and movements are contraindicated. Follow this flowchart to work out the programme that's right for you.

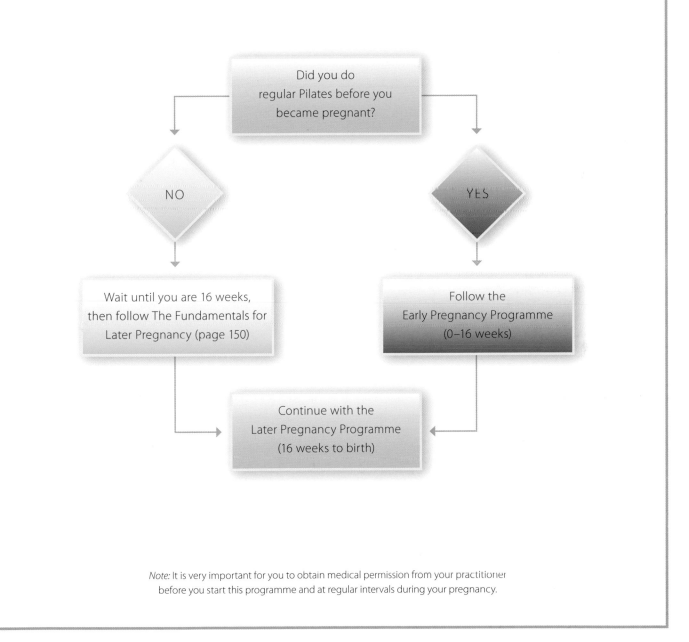

Did you do regular Pilates before you became pregnant?

NO

YES

Wait until you are 16 weeks, then follow The Fundamentals for Later Pregnancy (page 150)

Follow the Early Pregnancy Programme (0–16 weeks)

Continue with the Later Pregnancy Programme (16 weeks to birth)

Note: It is very important for you to obtain medical permission from your practitioner before you start this programme and at regular intervals during your pregnancy.

Your Changing Body (and How Pilates Can Help)

The maternal organs

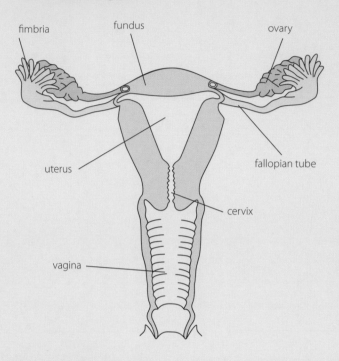

fimbria

fundus

ovary

uterus

fallopian tube

cervix

vagina

The pelvic organs

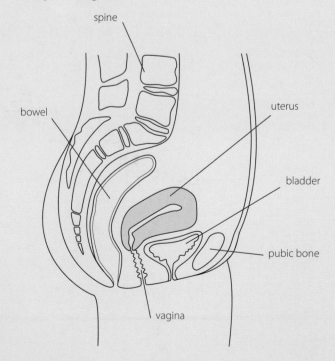

spine

bowel

uterus

bladder

pubic bone

vagina

Being aware of yourself and the many changes that will be taking place as your baby grows within you is very important, not just for your Pilates practice but for your health and self-awareness. Understanding your body will help you appreciate the miracle of motherhood, and, armed with this knowledge, allow you to better manage those changes.

The three trimesters

Pregnancies normally last about 40 weeks from conception to delivery although the range of 38–42 weeks is considered full term. Pregnancy is divided into three trimesters:

First trimester	0–12 weeks
Second trimester	13–26 weeks
Third trimester	27–40 weeks

As noted, our antenatal exercise programme has been divided into two parts. Early Pregnancy (0–16 weeks) and Later Pregnancy (16–40) weeks, so if you have been following the Early Pregnancy programme or if you are new to the programme, you would start the Later Pregnancy Programme 4 weeks into your second trimester.

What is happening inside?

When you are not pregnant, your uterus is a small, hollow, pear-shaped organ measuring about 8 x 5 x 2.5cm. It is a pelvic organ situated inside your abdominal cavity and lodged between the bladder in front and the rectum behind. Your abdominal cavity itself extends from your diaphragm (the large mushroom-shaped breathing muscle), beneath your lungs down to the muscles of your pelvic floor. Your uterus is a muscular organ, comprising a network of muscle fibres running in all directions.

The top part of the uterus is called the fundus, extending out from each side are the two fallopian tubes and these narrow canals end in finger-shaped projections called fimbria. The fimbria surround your ovaries and receive the ripe ovum (egg) after you ovulate. At the other end of the uterus is the cervix, which projects into the vagina. The cervix remains closed during pregnancy; the narrow opening is about 4cm long and is sealed with a mucous plug. During labour the cervix will need to open to about 10cm to allow your baby to be born, but we are getting ahead of ourselves...

Your baby is conceived in one of the fallopian tubes. While you might keep a diary of your activities, it's hard to say for sure when exactly sperm met egg so we count week 1 from the first day of your last menstrual period. Now starts the miraculous transformation from a single cell to your new child. The future baby makes its journey from the fallopian tube to the uterus and this embryo settles into the uterine lining which will be its home for the next 9 months (give or take). Meanwhile the amniotic sac, the bag of waters, is forming. This fluid will grow from a teaspoon's worth to 750ml by the time of the birth. This is your baby's protection from trauma and infection.

By your due date your uterus will have increased 5–6 times in size, 20 times in weight, stretched by your growing baby. At 16 weeks the fundus is nearly halfway to the navel, at 18 weeks it reaches the navel, at 36 weeks it lies just below the diaphragm. Two to 4 weeks before the birth the baby's presenting part may descend in readiness for the birth.

Your baby, snug in its new environment, is connected from the navel by an umbilical cord to the placenta, which is in turn attached to the wall of your uterus. The placenta will nourish your baby from your bloodstream while eliminating waste products back to you. Normally the placenta is situated in the upper segment of the uterus at the back, but sometimes it is implanted in front or lower down. Your baby has its own blood circulation system, blood flowing around its body through the umbilical cord, to the placenta and back again. The umbilical cord is therefore its lifeline. It will be severed only when the baby is born and breathing on their own.

The changing uterus

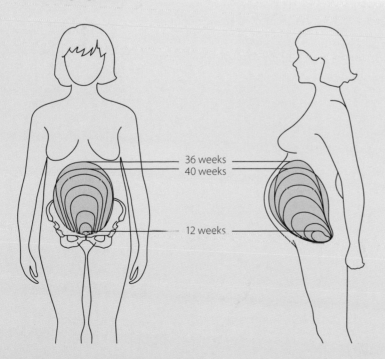

36 weeks
40 weeks

12 weeks

A baby at term

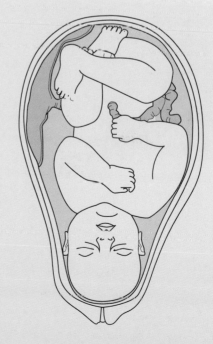

Hormonal influences on the body's systems

Buckle up and get ready for the ride of your life, because your body is going on a rollercoaster ride of hormonal change from the instant you become pregnant to weeks, if not months, after the birth of your baby.

These hormones trigger the changes that will make your body adapt in order to accommodate and nourish the growing baby. They get you ready for the delivery itself and for breastfeeding after the birth. The body releases a cocktail of pregnancy hormones, including extra progesterone, oestrogen and relaxin. These hormones will have an effect on all the body's organ systems. Let's look at some of the ways your body is changing and how regular Pilates can help.

We will start with breathing. The purpose of breathing is to transport a regular and plentiful supply of newly oxygenated blood around the body, delivering the vital nutrients needed to repair and grow and to clear away the waste products or toxins from your system. Taking a breath is the first thing we do, and the last. And yet most of us rarely give it a moment's thought. Most of us breathe far too quickly and too shallowly and end up using only a fraction of our capacity, decreasing our supply of oxygen and missing out on the vitality it brings.

Now when you are pregnant, you are not just breathing for one but two! So it makes even more sense to make sure that you are breathing as efficiently as possible. This is one of the many benefits doing Pilates regularly can bring. You will understand this better if you understand breathing and ways that the process can be made more efficient.

We breathe oxygen-rich air in through the nose, where tiny hairs filter out germs and dust particles. The air is warmed as it passes through the nasal passages on its way to the lungs. The oxygen molecules then pass from the lungs into the bloodstream where they are transported to the billions of cells within the body by the cardiovascular system. Simultaneously, carbon dioxide molecules produced as a waste product by the cells are transported to the lungs by the cardiovascular system where they pass from the bloodstream to the lungs. As we breathe out we expel the carbon dioxide-rich air from the lungs.

The lungs themselves do not contain any muscles, they simply expand into the empty space around them, known as the thoracic cavity. The lungs are surrounded by a strong membrane connecting them with the chest walls, the movements of which cause the lungs to expand and contract as we breathe in and out. The muscles involved in breathing are primarily the diaphragm and the intercostal muscles which lie between the ribs. The diaphragm is a double dome-shaped muscle, separating the thoracic cavity from the abdominal cavity. As well as being involved in breathing, the diaphragm is also responsible for increasing intra-abdominal pressure for stability and the evacuation of abdominal contents during defecation, urination, vomiting and yes, you've guessed it, childbirth!

The muscles used in the breathing process also have a role in posture, stability and movement (to be explored later in the book). Posture and breathing are closely connected. Your posture is going to affect the efficiency of your breathing. If your posture is poor, your shoulders are rounded, your ribs may be compressed and the space in the thoracic cavity is limited, thus your breathing may be impaired. So slouching is not only bad for your posture but also your breathing. Poor posture may disturb the flow of blood and thus disturb its efficiency at transporting oxygen and nutrients, as well as clearing away the toxins.

Take a deep breath in and notice how your abdomen expands. This is the diaphragm flattening out, moving down, so pressure in the abdomen increases. Now breathe out and notice how the abdomen relaxes back down as the diaphragm moves back up and the pressure in the abdomen decreases. This gentle rhythm is very beneficial, giving your internal organs a massage. We will be using this action later in the book to help you relax during labour and even to help you relax your pelvic floor!

When you become pregnant, there are some subtle changes to how you breathe. While your rate of respiration remains about the same, the depth of your respiration increases. There is a 15–20 per cent increase in oxygen consumption in pregnancy. Mild breathlessness is common. You may feel short of breath with even a little exercise. With your growing body weight, more oxygen is required to exercise. The hormones swell all the capillaries in the body, including those in the lungs and bronchial tubes, making it harder for you to catch your breath. Your diaphragm elevates, as do your ribs. Your hormones signal this change even before the ribs are squeezed up and out by the expanding uterus. As your baby grows, your lungs get crowded out. Do not worry, the baby is receiving plenty of oxygen. Though of course if you are really struggling to breathe, call for an ambulance.

We have described above the passage of air on its way to your lungs. Now your pregnancy hormones will also affect your respiratory tract. The increased blood flow associated with pregnancy swells the mucous membranes, increasing the amount of mucus, which can give you the symptoms of cold, sneezing and coughing (once again placing further strain on your pelvic floor). Nose bleeds are a common problem, but do mention them to your practitioner.

We will be discussing breathing again later in the chapter on The Fundamentals and in the chapter on Preparation for the Birth. But pregnancy is the perfect time to learn how to maximise your breath. You will be learning how to use your breathing to help your movements during your Pilates practice. And also how focusing on your breathing can help to calm your mind and body, which will prove invaluable when preparing for pregnancy, throughout your pregnancy, during labour and for precious relaxation once you've had your baby.

What else will be changing in your body?

Depending on the size of your baby, and how many you are having, your blood volume will progressively increase 30–50 per cent throughout the pregnancy, returning to normal 6–8 weeks after the birth. Your body must ensure that enough blood is pumped to and from the uterus and placenta, as well as supplying all your needs. This increase in volume puts added pressure on the blood vessels and would cause the blood pressure to rise, were it not for the relaxing hormonal effect on the vessels.

Your practitioner will be keeping a close eye on your blood pressure, checking it at each visit. The blood pressure usually dips in the first trimester, reaches its lowest level halfway through the pregnancy and then starts to climb, reaching its pre-pregnancy level about 6 weeks after the birth. Pilates, with its gentle, slow controlled movements, will be ideal for you. But you are going to need to take your time moving between exercises, avoiding any positions that make you feel dizzy or light-headed (see page 146 for how to get down and up safely from the floor).

All this extra blood needs pumping around your body so your heart will increase in size as the pregnancy progresses. Your heart rate goes up 10–20 beats a minute. It should return to normal about 6 weeks after the birth. While Pilates exercises do not raise the heart rate enough to count as aerobic exercise, they do help the circulation. It is important to include some gentle cardiovascular exercise in addition to your Pilates workouts, but you should be careful not to raise your heart rate too high (see page 219).

The best position for cardiac output is lying on your left side as this is the position that places minimum pressure on the aorta. The worst position is lying flat on your back (supine) as from about 16 weeks onwards, the increased weight of the uterus and baby may compress the inferior vena cava. This affects the venous return and decreases

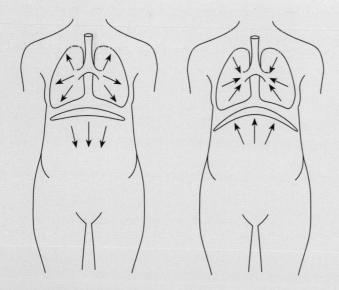

Inhalation as you breathe in, the diaphram moves down and pressure in the abdomen increases.

Exhalation as you breathe out, the diaphram moves up and pressure in the abdomen decreases.

cardiac output and may lead to a condition known as supine hypotensive syndrome, which we will be discussing at length later in the book (see page 136).

In addition to the increase in blood volume there is also an increase in fluid to all the body's tissues, including the lymphatic fluid, which is essentially the body's waste disposal system. As a result, fluid retention becomes a problem. Many Pilates exercises work on improving lymphatic drainage, which relies on muscular action, in the legs and thus help to keep those fluids moving.

Pregnant women may suffer from mild swelling of ankles and feet and sometimes hands and face – this is called oedema. As long as it is not excessive and there is no accompanying of raised blood pressure or protein in the urine it is considered normal. But oedema from the hips upwards, especially of the face, is monitored carefully as this may be the beginning of pre-eclampsia. Pre-eclampsia is a condition that can occur in pregnant women when there is a problem with the placenta (the organ that links the baby's blood supply to the mother's). The general rule of thumb is that if you have two of any of the following three symptoms then you will be monitored for pre-eclampsia: abdominal or facial swelling, protein in the urine (unless you have a urinary infection) and raised blood pressure.

In the first 12 weeks of pregnancy, the hormones also cause laxity of the arterial and venous walls, causing the blood pressure to go down. This may cause fainting and dizziness. You may also feel very tired as your blood volume goes up to accommodate the increased supply to the reproductive organs and placenta. This is known as haemo-dilution and makes the blood thin and watery. You may experience the symptoms of anaemia but you are not clinically anaemic as your iron levels are in fact normal (you just have more blood). By about week 16 you

> 'As a heavy rainstorm freshens the water of a stagnant stream and whips it into immediate action, so does the Pilates Method purify the blood stream.'
>
> *Joseph Pilates*

should start to feel more energetic. If you are feeling tired do mention this to your practitioner, who may suggest you take a supplement. Eating a healthy, balanced diet including iron-rich foods will help. Do not try to exercise if you feel tired. Learn to listen to when your body needs rest, not activity.

In a normal pregnancy one-sixth of your blood volume is within the uterine vascular system. An increase in kidney blood flow helps the removal of the metabolic waste created by your growing baby. Your hormones will have signalled an increase not just in blood flow but urine flow too as you have more urine to pass, yours and your baby's. And all at a time when your pelvic floor muscles are already under pressure! To make matters worse, the angle that the urethra enters the bladder alters because the uterus is enlarging. This can cause a reflux (backwash) of urine back into the urethra from the bladder where it may pool, making you prone to urinary tract infections. Try leaning forward to urinate as this helps empty the bladder completely. Don't be tempted to cut back on fluid intake during the day, but you can avoid too much before bedtime.

The pregnancy hormones will have relaxed the smooth muscle tissue everywhere in the body, and this includes the gastrointestinal tract. This tends to slow down the transit of food through the system, which can leave you with indigestion and feeling bloated. You may find that you are constipated. That's the bad news. The good news is that the extra transit time allows more time for nutrients to be absorbed into the bloodstream, where they travel to the placenta and thus to the baby.

Heartburn is another common antenatal condition as the muscle that separates the oesophagus from the stomach relaxes ,allowing the food and digestive juices to reflux from the stomach into the oesophagus, where they may irritate the lining. Bear this in mind when you plan the timing of your sessions. We have included some exercises which you might find helpful.

The pelvis and ligamentous laxity

If you have never thought about your pelvis before, now is the time! It's where much of the action is going to take place, so it needs a closer look.

Your pelvic girdle is a ring of bones. The large triangular bone at the back is the sacrum, consisting of fused vertebrae. The sacrum is connected to the coccyx (tailbone) at the sacrococcygeal joint. The two large pelvic bones are the ilium bones. They are connected to the sacrum at the back at the two sacroiliac joints and at the symphysis pubis at the front (the pubic bone). The ischia are the bones that you sit upon.

The symphysis pubis, sacroiliac and sacrococcygeal joints are held together with strong ligaments. Ligaments are strong fibrous bands of connective tissue. They are not normally pliable; normally they are non-elastic with all the flexibility of a piece of cotton! The cocktail of hormones released when you become pregnant softens these ligaments, increasing their elasticity, giving them a consistency more like a piece of lycra rather than cotton. Why?

Well, it's all to do with one of the most important journeys your baby will ever make (apart perhaps from its journey down the fallopian tube!). Your baby has to pass through your pelvis which is the shape of a curved funnel. Viewing the pelvis from above you can see the pelvic inlet – your baby's head will descend into this (engage), in readiness to be born and it will then, with a little help from you, pass through the pelvic outlet and into the world. To enable this to happen the ligaments have to be more elastic and allow the pelvis to expand. The sacroiliac joints will thus be allowed to expand to adapt to the shape of the baby's head. The sacrococcygeal joint can loosen and move out of the way as the baby is delivered.

This is important to remember as we are going to use this to our advantage in the exercise programme as we prepare for the birth. How are we going to do this? By getting into positions that encourage this opening. Try this experiment.

Stand up and place your hands on your ischia (sitting bones). Then squat down a little. Notice what happens to those sitting bones? They should move apart as you squat down. This creates more space for your baby to descend. This is why we will be practising lots and lots of squats!

The pelvic bones

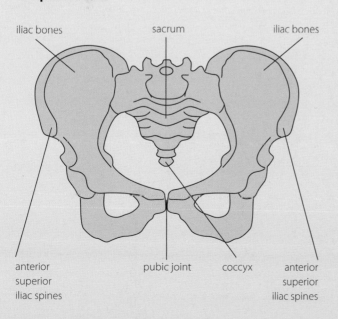

iliac bones   sacrum   iliac bones

anterior
superior   pubic joint   coccyx   anterior
iliac spines   superior
                                                  iliac spines

The pelvic canal

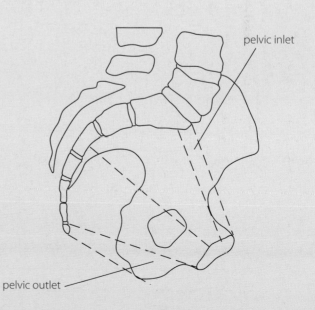

pelvic inlet

pelvic outlet

We have seen, therefore, why ligamentous laxity is essential. But it comes at a price. Sometimes it can cause pelvic girdle problems, especially if your pelvic muscles are not strong enough to give you adequate support or if you place undue strain on your joints. A lot of sacroiliac joint problems start during pregnancy or in the period after the birth. It is a similar case with pubis symphysis dysfunction; the joint here may even separate (a condition known as diastasis symphysis).

How can you ensure that you do not place unnecessary strain on your pelvic joints? You need to avoid positions and movements which load the pelvis unevenly. For example, we will be avoiding single leg weight-bearing exercises as this loads just one side of your pelvis and may cause problems. Similarly, we do not want to pull unequally on the muscles connected to the pelvis. In particular we are going to be very cautious with stretches. Let's take another look at the pelvic ligaments.

The two ligaments we are focusing on are the sacrotuberous ligament and the sacrospinous ligament. These two are important stabilising ligaments for the pelvis. The sacrotuberous ligament has attachments to the muscles at the back of the thighs (hamstrings).

The sacrospinous ligament has connections with the coccyx bone, pelvic floor and inner thigh muscles (adductors). If we pull on the hamstrings and adductors, especially if we pull unevenly on them, we risk destabilising the pelvic joints. With this in mind, when planning the exercise programme we have avoided any movements or positions that pull or strain on these joints. We will be explaining later in the chapter on The Fundamentals that in Pilates we usually use movement to achieve length in muscles rather than traditional stretching (see page 71). But if you do wish to stretch, be sure to apply the stretch evenly on both sides.

The symphysis pubis is another joint which can be made more vulnerable by the ligamentous laxity of pregnancy. We will therefore also avoid any position or movements that pull or strain on this joint.

That's what we are *not* going to do. What we are going to do is ensure that all the relevant muscles that support your pelvis are of adequate strength and length to do their role efficiently! The exercises are going to help you create your own girdle of support or corset to help prevent pelvic girdle pain (see page 193).

Strong ligaments hold the pelvic bones in place

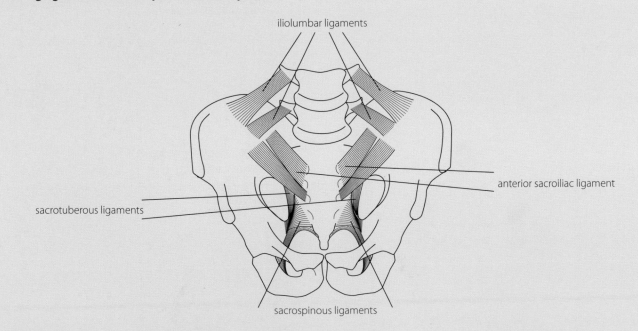

iliolumbar ligaments

anterior sacroiliac ligament

sacrotuberous ligaments

sacrospinous ligaments

Your posture in pregnancy

One of the most dramatic changes to your body over the nine months of pregnancy is to your posture. This isn't surprising. The extra weight you are carrying is mainly upfront. This is going to affect how you stand and how you move. Even if you normally have great posture you may find that it deteriorates with the added load on board.

What makes the impact even greater is the ligamentous laxity we have just discussed, as this may make all your joints more prone to instability, not just your pelvis – your knees, feet, ankles, shoulders. Your spine may be more dynamic. In short, your posture reacts much more than normal to the changes in weight distribution. The growing breasts and baby shift your centre of gravity upwards and forwards. Then in order for you to maintain your balance and stability, your posture has to compensate.

So exactly how will your posture change? That depends on a wide range of factors, almost too many to mention. So many things can influence posture. There are hereditary factors, environmental factors, sports and hobbies, the work you do, your nutrition, your mood... to name but a few. During pregnancy we can add to the list: the amount of give in your ligaments, your pre-pregnancy posture, the strength of your deep postural muscles, how much weight you gain, how many babies you are carrying, the size of your baby, the extent of your abdominal divide (the diastasis recti – see page 24), your postural awareness. All these can have an impact on your posture and movement patterns. As we have noted, no two mothers are the same and no two pregnancies the same. Just take a look at the pictures on page 21!

But we can identify two common compensations at either end of the scale. Let's call them Postures A and B. In the chapter on The Fundamentals, we have given you some guidelines on how to assess your own posture – it's not foolproof, but gives you some idea of how your posture is changing. Ideally you would check with your Pilates teacher or healthcare practitioner.

Posture A This is what is commonly regarded as a typical pregnancy posture. After about 12 weeks of pregnancy, the baby has grown and the uterus is too large to remain wholly within the pelvis and becomes an abdominal organ. This has an impact on the angle of your pelvis. In response to the growing bump, your pelvis tips to counterbalance the extra load; in the case of Posture A, the pelvis tips forward, thus increasing your lumbar curve (lordosis). If this is the case you will feel an increased hollow in your lower back. With your centre of gravity no longer falling through your feet, you may compensate by leaning back to correct this shift. This means that you are now weight-bearing through your lumbar spine, the facet joints, the posterior ligaments and the intervertebral discs. Your overloaded muscles then get tired very quickly especially if you have to stand or sit still for long.

Posture A (typical pregnancy posture)

Meanwhile, further up the spine, the increased weight of the growing breasts pulls the upper (thoracic) spine into a greater curvature (kyphosis). Your upper back becomes more rounded. This alters the angle of your head and neck and in order to see where you are going you have to thrust your head forward and tip it back, thus increasing the curve in your neck and shortening the back of the neck. It is very easy then for neck tension to creep in.

With a rounded upper back, your shoulder joints are now out of good alignment. Your arms tend to be rotated inwards at the shoulder joints, perhaps leaving you feeling tight across your chest. Your shoulder-blades may have shifted on the back of your ribcage, and moved upwards and outwards, resulting in important stabilising muscles being held in a lengthened position, reducing their ability to work properly. This can sometimes lead to shoulder-joint problems, which will be further exacerbated by all the forward bending involved in caring for your new baby.

If your pelvis has tilted forwards it can affect the angle and mobility of your hips. Perhaps you find yourself hyperextending your knees (locking your knees back.) Your thighbones may be rotated inwards, your shinbones rotated outwards, which in turn may affect your walking pattern. Your feet may pronate (roll inwards), this being further exacerbated by your lax ligaments and a possible drop in your arches. Weight shifts back towards your heels to bring the centre of gravity to a more posterior position. All this will help contribute towards the pregnancy 'waddle'.

Posture B In this posture, while your upper body may still have changed as described above, your pelvis has not tipped forwards to compensate for the growing baby and uterus but rather backwards, thus decreasing your lumbar curve. This may put an increased strain on where your lumbar spine meets the back of your pelvis, the large triangular bone which is the sacrum. The joints at the back of your pelvis (your sacroiliac joints) are now carrying extra load. Your lumbar spine appears flatter than normal. So, rather than an increased hollow in your lower back you will feel a reduced hollow. As before, your centre of gravity has shifted.

These postural changes do not automatically mean that you will get back pain or joint problems, but they may be a contributory factor. A lot of women report that their back problems first started during pregnancy. If nothing is done, these problems do not always automatically disappear after the birth and can go on to be long-term problems. If you experience back or other joint pain, do talk to your medical practitioner. They may refer you to a physiotherapist, osteopath or chiropractor. Once you have been cleared to exercise, Pilates can help enormously by improving your postural awareness, your muscular control and strength.

Posture B

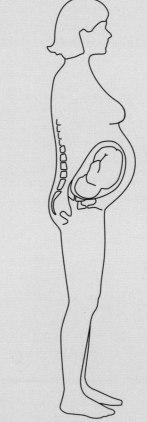

Different pregnancy postures

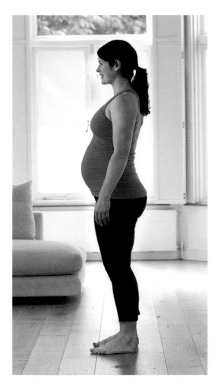
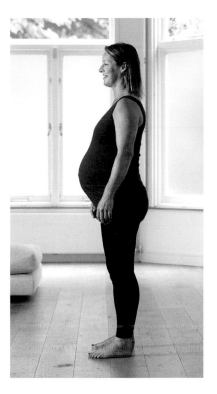
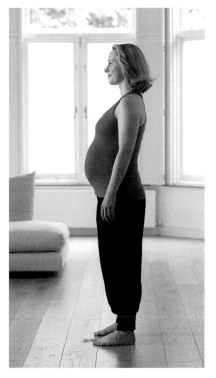
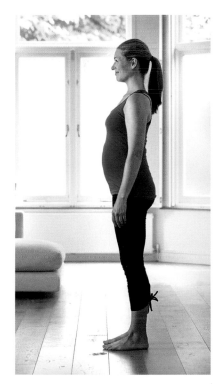
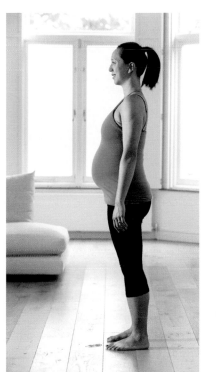
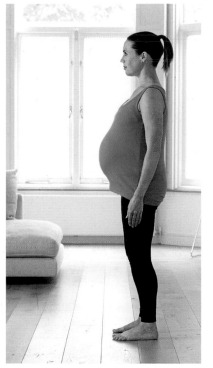

Good postural alignment will help the forces of gravity be more evenly distributed through your body. There should be less overload, less wear and tear on your joint structures and the natural balance and correct length of your muscles is maintained, enabling them to function more efficiently.

In The Fundamentals we shall be giving you guidelines on how to achieve better posture. But to facilitate any lasting changes to posture and movement you need to understand and experience how to use your body well so that it becomes habitual. Being aware of good posture is important not just in your Pilates practice, but in your daily activities, to notice when you are slouching or waddling! See page 142 for advice on this.

Furthermore, awareness of good alignment is only half the battle. You need to develop your ability to maintain good alignment and control your movements. Posture is not a static thing, it's dynamic. Even if we think we are standing still, our muscles and our nerves are in fact making hundreds of small adjustments every second in response to the pull of gravity and our surroundings. Good posture requires strength and endurance in these deep postural muscles. For good posture and movement to be habitual, you have to pattern your movements and this means practice, practice, practice. You need good movement to be ingrained in your body.

Good posture in pregnancy

Notice the points of the body through which the imaginary plumbline falls:
– The ear lobe
– The bodies of the cervical vertebrae (the neck)
– The tip of the shoulder
– Dividing the thorax (ribcage) in half
– The bodies of the lumbar vertebrae
– Slightly behind the hip joint
– Slightly in front of the centre of the knee joint
– Slightly in front of the outside ankle bone
(lateral malleolus)

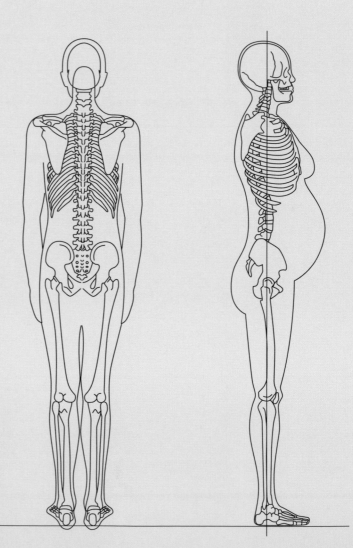

Your natural corset

How would you like a natural, in-built, go with you everywhere, all the time, corset? One that enables you to still breathe, that doesn't bulge, ride up or give you visible panty lines? Well, the exercises in this book can give you such a girdle! In fact, Pilates is famous for exactly this.

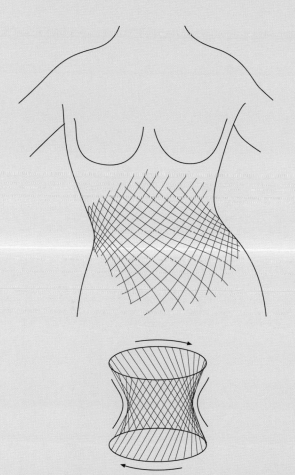

What do we mean by a natural girdle?

You have several layers of abdominal muscles starting with the most superficial layer, the rectus abdominis (commonly known as the six-pack muscle), the external and internal obliques and the deepest layer of all, the transversus abdominis, the fibres of which wrap horizontally across your torso.

Core cylinder

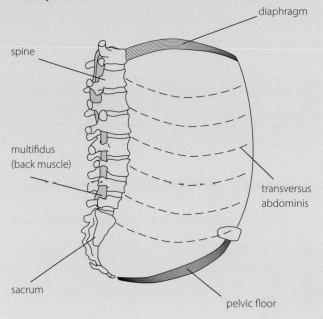

Depending on the movement you are doing or the position you are in, each set of muscles has a different role to play. All are important. The transversus muscle, for example, is not a movement muscle but rather one that, together with other deep core muscles (notably the deep spinal muscles, diaphragm and pelvic floor), plays a supportive role for your pelvis and spine. It will also support your growing uterus and baby.

This muscle is involved in the delivery of your baby, when the time comes. The beauty of a Pilates workout is that you are training these very muscles every time you do an exercise. The principle of Centring, working from a stable centre, lies at the heart of Pilates and will be discussed later on pages 58–59.

All these abdominal muscles will be affected by your pregnancy hormones. They will become more pliable. This is to allow the abdominals to stretch and accommodate your growing bump, which may reduce their ability to support your lower back and pelvis. The rectus abdominis is going to divide along its centre line, the linea alba, so that your bump can grow. This separation is called diastasis recti.

Diastasis recti

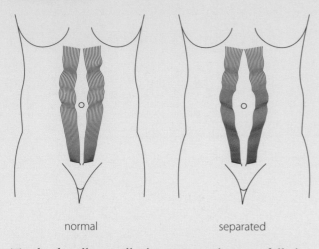

normal   separated

The divide will normally close again, perhaps not fully, but to within 2cm width after the birth, which is considered normal. Unfortunately, sometimes this divide is wider than expected – for example if the mother is having twins, a large baby, or has had multiple pregnancies. It may not improve even after the birth. The divide can prove problematic as it may reduce the ability of the abdominal muscles to control the pelvis and the spine and increases the risk of a herniation.

Notice how the separation of the muscle has changed the angle in which the fibres run. This is the muscle responsible for trunk flexion (for example Curl Ups on page 72). With the separation the muscles pull at a different angle. We do not wish to strengthen these muscles in this altered position. This is why we do not recommend any curl-up style exercises from 16 weeks onwards. We will be discussing this at greater length in the chapter on After the Birth (page 188) but we have taken this into account when choosing which exercises to do throughout the pregnancy.

For our girdle to give us enough support, we need to work on building strength from the inside out. We need to create a strong and stable foundation. We will be doing this right through the programme from Preparing for Pregnancy through to our Postnatal Programme with all the exercises for pelvic and spinal stability. These are going to prove valuable for helping to prevent the divide from becoming too wide.

The bottom line: the importance of your pelvic floor

As your baby grows there is going to be increased weight on your pelvic floor muscles. What do we mean by the pelvic floor?

The pelvic floor consists of three muscles – pubococcygeus, iliococcygeus, ischicoccygeus. As their names suggest they connect the pubic bone at the front to the coccyx (tailbone) and the ischial tuberosities (your sitting bones) at the back. It's a misnomer really to call it a pelvic floor as these muscles are slanted at different angles and layers and do not form a 'floor' at all. These muscles support all the pelvic contents, the uterus, bladder and bowels. Together they form a figure of eight around the vagina and anus.

Their situation gives them a vital support role, especially when you are carrying the extra load of a growing uterus and baby. If you had to carry a cardboard box full of heavy bottles, how would you carry it? Would you hold just the sides of the box? Of course not, you would support it from underneath. This is why we will be teaching you how to engage the pelvic floor along with your abdominals when you connect to your core (see page 60).

Pelvic floor muscles

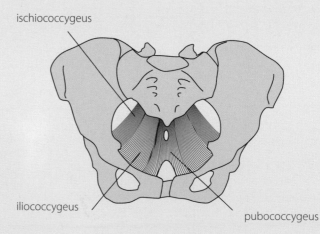

ischiococcygeus

iliococcygeus   pubococcygeus

Pelvic floor at rest and engaged

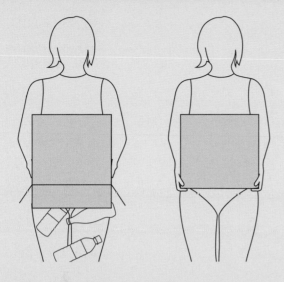

These are the muscles that can help prevent you leaking urine when you cough or sneeze or jump. Owning up to having pelvic floor problems is not always an easy thing for a woman to do (even harder for a man). So many women suffer in silence, but it's a very common problem and help is at hand. Talk to your doctor, who may then decide to refer you to a woman's health physiotherapist (misnamed as they also help men).

Pelvic floor problems may be caused by a variety of reasons. Sometimes it is an unfortunate combination of causes. If the muscles have been strained they will weaken. For example if you repeatedly lift heavy loads, or cough excessively; if you are constipated and strain when evacuating your bowels. Hormones influence these muscles not just in pregnancy but later in life when you are going through the menopause. But the obvious culprit is childbirth, especially if you have a prolonged second stage of labour with a lot of pushing, a large or awkwardly positioned baby, deep tearing, or complications leading to medical interventions such as the use of forceps and episiotomies (see page 172).

Even if you have a caesarean section you may not avoid pelvic floor problems. You have still been carrying the baby for nine months. As the uterus becomes heavier, it is the pelvic floor that must bear the weight. It may drop as much as 2.5cm, not to mention the fact that towards the end the baby, as already mentioned, is likely to use the pelvic floor just like a trampoline!

So gaining control over your pelvic floor muscles can help with a wide range of ante- and postnatal problems such as urinary and faecal incontinence. Pelvic floor exercises can also improve circulation to the pelvic area, helping to improve the functioning of the reproductive organs and helping to prevent haemorrhoids. This improved circulation will also aid the healing process after the birth itself. And let's be honest, good pelvic floor control enhances sexual enjoyment too so may even be said to have a role to play in preparing for a baby!

But notice that we have been talking about pelvic floor control rather than strength. These are muscles like any other muscles and to work properly they need the appropriate amount of tone and length. They are designed to stretch so that your baby can come out, but you will need to learn how to release them. In this way you may be able to prevent tearing or having to have an episiotomy during the delivery. It is also important to be able to release your pelvic floor even when you are not pregnant to help avoid over-activity in these muscles.

So now you know why we have included a lot of pelvic floor education in all the exercise programmes!

The pelvic floor trampoline

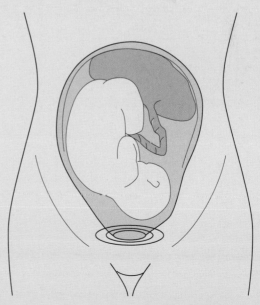

Relaxation, mental and emotional health

If your hormones are giving you a physical rollercoaster of a ride, consider too the rollercoaster of emotions and feelings associated with preparing for pregnancy, pregnancy itself and the pressures of motherhood. Expect mood swings, irrational behaviour, high levels of irritability and anxiety! It is easy enough to say avoid becoming stressed, but much harder to do. You may be worrying about a host of things: your ability to become pregnant, your changing body, worrying if the baby is okay, will you be able to cope with labour and the delivery, with motherhood? Add to all these worries a heady cocktail of hormones and no wonder you are prone to feeling weepy and fragile!

It is worth remembering that stress itself is not a bad thing. It is the natural response to danger, the fight or flight defence our ancestors needed for survival. Our adrenal glands release cortisol and adrenalin to give us the sudden burst of energy we need to run from the charging woolly mammoth! We might not need to run from the mammoth these days but we have different challenges with money and employment worries, marital problems and so on. While you might be tempted to run away from your last heating bill, the problems we face nowadays are not so easy to deal with immediately. This often means that we do not come back down from the fight or flight stress response and may remain in a state of stress which can be negative to our wellbeing and the baby's health.

The 'feel-good' endorphins that are released naturally after any type of exercise play a valuable role in keeping your spirits high and in giving you self-confidence. It feels good to keep active. After doing an exercise session the level of cortisol in your body drops significantly – leaving you feeling calmer.

Taking time out to relax and simply 'be' can be enormously beneficial. A gentle stroll can work wonders. If you haven't tried meditation, do give it a go as it is a wonderful way to control your stress levels and perfect for pregnancy. But if you are someone who finds traditional meditation difficult, you may find that thoughtful, mindful exercise like Pilates or yoga does the trick.

The release of tension in the body is a starting point for Pilates. It is one of our guiding principles. Pilates will also give you awareness of the breath, help to clear your mind and bring you into the moment. It can be like a meditation through movement.

Learning to release unwanted tension is going to be a useful tool before, during and after your pregnancy. Bear in mind too that anxiety and stress are not helpful when you are trying to conceive. In the first few months of your pregnancy, your body must focus on building the baby's life support system so you need to conserve your energy and rest. Not always easy if you are used to being on the go all the time. As the months go by, you will need to plan some relaxation time into your schedule. Quiet time to bond with your unborn baby. Relaxation can help with hypertension (high blood pressure), back problems and indigestion. Then there's the labour itself, which can go on for many hours. If you remain in a state of tension, you can be exhausted by the birth itself, you may even be too tired to push! Pilates can teach you to use the breath to release tension, to control movement and to breathe through discomfort.

And then, once your new baby is born, you will need to make the most of rare moments of peace. Relaxation may also help with breastfeeding. A baby can easily sense if its mother or father, are stressed. This relaxation time is essential particularly if you have other children to look after, are working and/or have very little time for yourself.

But learning to relax takes practice. Thus, we have included plenty of 'release' exercises in the programme, as well as specific Relaxation exercises. Use your Pilates sessions as time to reflect, to bond with your unborn baby, to find inner calm and harmony.

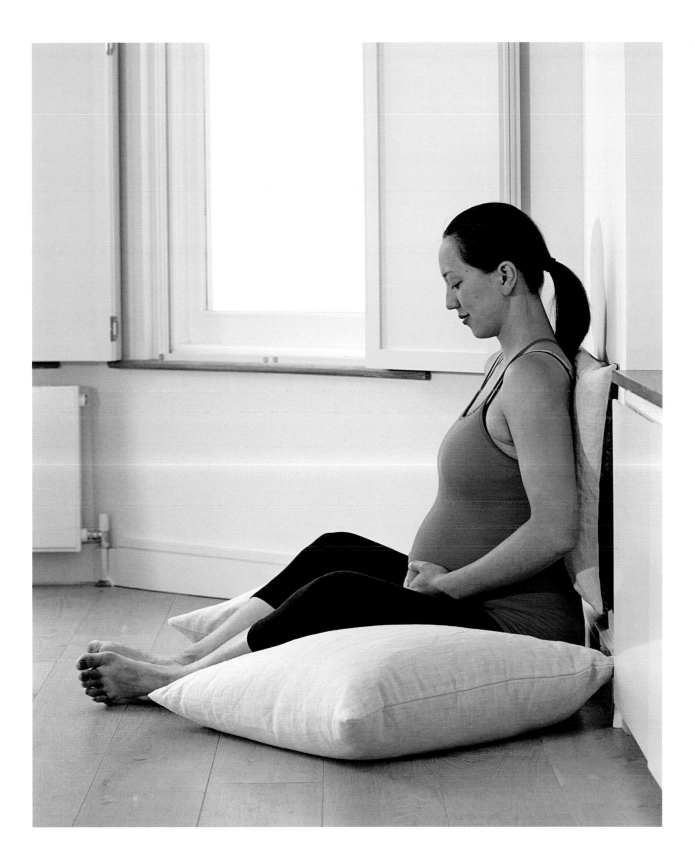

Before You Begin

Always prepare the space in which you are going to exercise by making it warm, comfortable and free from distractions. Make sure that you have enough room to move your arms and legs without knocking any ornaments off the coffee table. If you like, you can play some background music, but it should be quiet and not distracting!

Wear clothing that allows for freedom of movement, especially around the hips.

Gather together everything that you are going to need before you start. As your pregnancy progresses, you will need lots of additional support in the way of pillows and cushions.

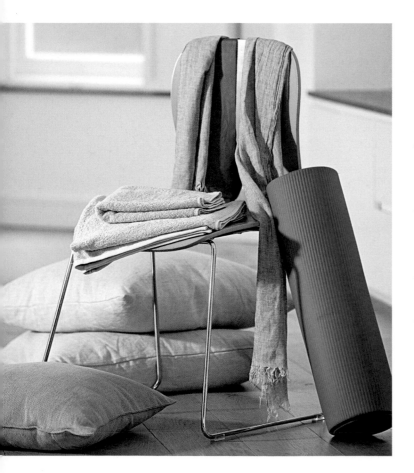

Equipment you are going to need

∗   Non-slip mat

∗   A folded towel or small flat pillow

∗   At least 3 plump pillows

∗   Stretch band (medium strength) or a long stretchy scarf

∗   Medium sized towel (for the postnatal programme)

∗   Sturdy chair without arms

∗   Some clear wall space

Do not exercise if:

∗   You are feeling unwell or tired

∗   You have just eaten a heavy meal

∗   You have been drinking alcohol

∗   You are in pain from injury. Always consult your practitioner first, as rest may be needed before exercise.

∗   You are undergoing medical treatment or are taking medication. Again, you will need to consult your practitioner first.

When is it not safe to exercise?

The exercises in this book are designed for women who are preparing for pregnancy, are having a normal pregnancy, or are postnatal with no complications. There are certain contraindications to exercise in pregnancy, listed below. But it is impossible to list all the contraindications which is why you must visit your practitioner to obtain permission to follow this programme. Do remember that your condition and ability to exercise may change.

Definite contraindications to exercise in pregnancy are:

∗   Three or more miscarriages

∗   Maternal heart disease

∗   Maternal diabetes

* Pain
* Bleeding
* High blood pressure
* Fever
* If you suffer from severe headaches, especially if they are accompanied by swelling, blurring of vision or pain at the side of the ribcage as these symptoms could indicate pre-eclampsia. See your GP immediately.
* Incompetent cervix
* Placenta praevia – as the placenta may detach before the pregnancy reaches full term
* If you are having twins, seek medical advice as to whether you may follow this programme.
* The following guidelines relate to cardiovascular exercise, but if you suffer from any of the following you may be advised by your doctor not to do Pilates exercise:
  – Severe anaemia
  – Cardiac arrhythmia
  – Chronic bronchitis
  – Type 1 diabetes
  – Morbid obesity
  – Extreme underweight
  – Intrauterine growth restriction in current pregnancy
  – Orthopaedic limitations
  – Poorly controlled seizure disorder
  – Poorly controlled thyroid disease
  – Heavy smoking

The risk of miscarriage

One in four pregnancies end in miscarriage; sadly it is very common. The first three months, and in particular the period 8–14 weeks, is the period when most miscarriages occur so this is a time for caution. Ultimately the decision whether to continue exercising or not rests with you and your doctor. We can only offer general advice. If you are at all apprehensive, then wait until after 16 weeks when the pregnancy is well established.

When to stop exercising

If at any time during the pregnancy you experience any of the following, do not continue with the exercises and immediately seek medical advice:

* If your membranes have ruptured
* If you are in pain
* If you are bleeding or leaking fluid
* If you are very short of breath
* If you feel dizzy, faint and/or disorientated
* If you develop tachycardia – fast heartbeat or an irregular heartbeat
* If you have pubic pain
* If you have difficulty in walking
* If your blood pressure is high
* If you develop severe headaches accompanied by swelling, blurring of vision, pain at the side of the ribcage; all indicate immediate referral to GP (could indicate pre-eclampsia)
* If you are unwell or have fever
* If you are very anaemic
* If you develop phlebitis (vein inflammation)
* If you have a breech in your third trimester, seek advice. Sometimes exercise is used to turn the baby but you will need medical guidance as to which exercises are suitable.
* If you haven't felt the baby move – you should feel at least ten movements per 12 waking hours. In the second trimester the baby's movements will be quite vigorous but in the third trimester when they have less space to move, the movements will feel more like he/she is squirming.
* If your pulse stays elevated after exercise
* If you develop swelling, pain or tenderness in calf or leg, there is a chance you may have developed a deep vein thrombosis.

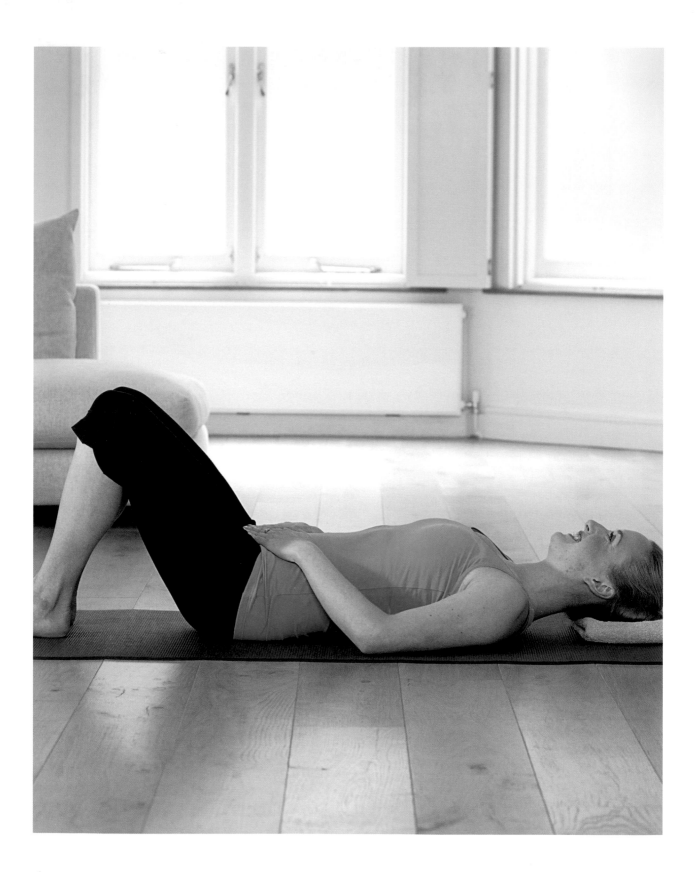

1

Learning the Fundamentals of Pilates

The Fundamentals of Body Control Pilates

This the most important chapter of the book as it contains all the basic skills you will need to perform the exercises well. Even if you are a Pilates veteran you should revisit The Fundamentals regularly to ensure good practice and keep up to date with the latest medical advice.

Take your time to read through this section carefully and learn each new exercise before moving onto the next. In this way you will be able to integrate each new skill into your practice, each skill like a building block. The basic skills form the foundation of good technique and ensure that you get maximum results. Attempting Pilates without due attention to these Fundamentals would be like building a house on sand!

Be prepared to find it all a bit confusing at first. At first you may find it daunting – keeping alignment, breathing, and connecting to your core – but eventually it all comes together and becomes natural. You will need time and practice, as the many changes happening to your body while pregnant can make this task even more challenging. Be patient. Practice makes perfect.

The basic skills you will need to begin are the ABCs of Alignment, Breathing and Centring (stability/mobility).

Alignment

Exercising with your body in good alignment is at the heart of good Pilates. As your pregnancy progresses, we will need to look at changing the normal exercise positions for some exercises so that you are not lying flat on your back, to avoid possible supine hypotensive syndrome (page 136). It is important that you experiment with the different variations shown to find which suits you best.

In this section we will be looking at ways to help you recognise good alignment in a variety of positions. You will need to learn how to find the right starting and finishing positions for the exercises, as well as controlling your alignment while performing the movements themselves. Good alignment relates to how you position the body both while you are 'still' and when you are moving. The reason alignment ranks so high on our list of priorities is because, if your body is habitually out of good alignment, it places an enormous strain on your joints, ligaments, muscles and has a detrimental effect on how you move.

This is mind and body training at its best and will help improve your overall posture and movements in everyday life.

During your pregnancy, and for several months after, your posture is changing quite dramatically. The increased weight of the baby and uterus, the increased size and weight of your breasts, your overall weight gain, the ligamentous laxity, the change in your centre of gravity… all these things mean that maintaining good postural alignment is even more vital.

In addition, you may find that your hormones have affected your spatial awareness. With this in mind, we will take time here to explain each different Starting position and for each one you will also see Watchpoints to help you perform the exercises even better. We've done everything we can to help you in the absence of us being in the room with you!

Details count! How you place your hands, feet, head, neck and shoulders while doing the exercises will all contribute to good posture. Pay close attention to the directions given in each exercise. A misplaced foot may prevent your pelvis from being in the right position. A tilted head may contribute to neck tension. Also, good hand, wrist, elbow and shoulder alignment may help prevent conditions such as carpal tunnel syndrome.

Let's look first at the spinal alignment. The vertebral

column consists of 24 flexible vertebrae, which are classified into three regions related to their function and structure: cervical (neck), thoracic (upper spine attached to the ribs) and lumbar (lower spine). The natural curves of the spine develop during early childhood and enable the spine to absorb some of the shock that would otherwise be transmitted up to our head when we move. When we stand, the deep postural muscles of the body are working constantly to keep us upright. One of the benefits of doing Pilates regularly is that you strengthen these deep postural muscles. As a result, standing tall with good postural alignment becomes easier.

Any change in the curves of one part of the spine will have an impact on the other curves. If you habitually sit slumped in a chair, you alter the angles of the curves of the spine, which may stress the ligaments, muscles and intervertebral discs. This is why it is important to be aware of your posture in your daily activities (see page 142).

The natural curves of the spine

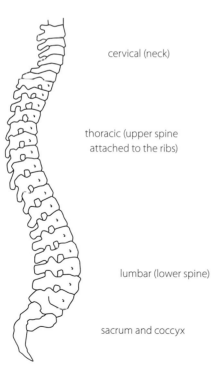

cervical (neck)

thoracic (upper spine attached to the ribs)

lumbar (lower spine)

sacrum and coccyx

We are aiming for a spine that is able to retain its natural curves, an elongated S-shape. There are many forces that conspire to compress our spine on a daily basis, including gravity, poor posture and in pregnancy the weight of the growing uterus and baby. We are going to try to limit these effects by creating more space between the vertebrae, so you will find we give the direction 'lengthen the spine' frequently in the exercises.

The angle of the pelvis will have an impact on the curvature of the spine. If you tilt your pelvis backwards, moving the pubic bone forward and tucking your tailbone under, you will lose some, if not all, of the hollow curve (lordosis) of your lumbar spine. If you tilt your pelvis forwards, moving the pubic bone backwards, you will increase the hollow of your lumbar spine.

But of course much depends on your normal posture and where your spine and pelvis are to start with! What we are looking for ideally is a comfortable mid, balanced, or ' neutral' position between these two extremes. The Compass exercise (see page 42) helps you find neutral.

When the pelvis is in neutral, the pubic bone and the prominent pelvic bones (anterior superior iliac spines) are level, which means that the pelvis is neither tipped too far forward (anteriorly) or back (posteriorly). Also the prominent pelvic bones should be level with each other, the waist equal in length on both sides. Neutral should eventually feel natural and comfortable – it is not a fixed point to be held at all costs!

What is important to remember is that each and every body is different. This is why we need to start with looking at your own posture. We also need to remember that your posture will change as your pregnancy progresses. Similarly, once you have had your baby your posture may change again. It would be very helpful if you revisit the following Assessment at regular intervals.

Assessing your Posture

To assess your posture we are going to use a wall because it will give you some feedback. Initially, do not alter your posture at all – just take note of where everything is. Stand with your back against a wall. Have your heels a comfortable distance (up to 30cm) away from the wall.

Notice the following:

✻ Where is your head in relation to the wall? Do not tip your head back, but allow the head to balance freely on top of your spine. Unless you have a very upright posture it is unlikely that the back of the head will touch the wall.

✻ Notice which parts of your upper spine touch the wall.

✻ Can you feel your shoulder-blades resting against the wall?

✻ Notice if your lumbar spine touches the wall. Is there a gap there? Notice how large that gap is by slipping the flat of your hand behind your waist.

✻ Can you feel the back of your pelvis, in particular the sacrum (the large triangular bone at the back of the pelvis) touching the wall?

So what have you discovered?

Let's focus on the lumbar curve first. While it is normal to have a small curve in the lumbar spine, we do not want this curve to be excessive.

✻ If you felt a gap of more than a hand's depth, we will call your posture Posture A. You would benefit enormously from practising Wall Slides Variation A (see page 36) on a regular basis. In fact we recommend that you start your Pilates workouts with Wall Slides as it will help to bring your spine and pelvis into better alignment.

✻ If you only felt a small gap in the lumbar spine (perhaps you could only just slide your hand in or not at all) we will call your posture Posture B. You will find Wall Slides Variation B useful.

Posture A

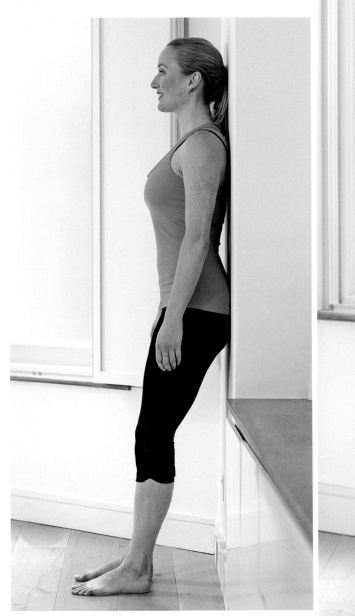

Notice how large the gap is between the wall and your lumbar spine by slipping the flat of your hand behind your waist.

Posture B

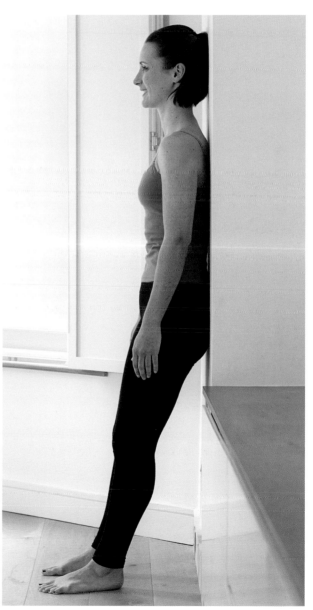

Wall Slides Variation A

Suitable for... All stages. Particularly valuable if you are Posture A, that is, if you have an increased lumbar hollow. **Aim** To develop awareness of your own individual posture and help improve your alignment.

Starting position...
Stand about 30cm away from a wall. Lean back into the wall. Have your feet hip-width apart and parallel. Knees bent a little.

✱ Watchpoints

– When you have learnt how to engage your core muscles, use them to help roll the pelvis and support your spine.

– Rather than simply pressing your back into the wall, think instead of gently opening, lengthening and imprinting the back.

– Be aware of the effect this movement is having on the rest of your body.

– Stay open and released across the shoulders.

– Do not tip your head back onto the wall. If it does not naturally rest on the wall allow it to balance freely on top of the spine.

– Keep your feet grounded, press the floor away evenly through both feet.

Action...

1 Breathe in to prepare your body to move. (If you like you can place your hands onto your pelvis so that you can feel what's happening.)

2 Breathe out and gently roll your pelvis backwards, your pubic bone curls forward, so that your low back lengthens and flattens against the wall.

3 Breathe in, then as you breathe out slide down the wall a few centimetres. Try to keep your tailbone on the wall. Imagine you are imprinting your low back into the wall.

4 Breathe in and slowly start to straighten you legs while keeping your low back against the wall. Stop when you start to feel that your low back has come away from the wall. **Repeat** *up to 8 times, by which time, hopefully your pelvis and spine have been encouraged to be in a mid neutral position. When you step away from the wall, try to remember this new lengthened position.*

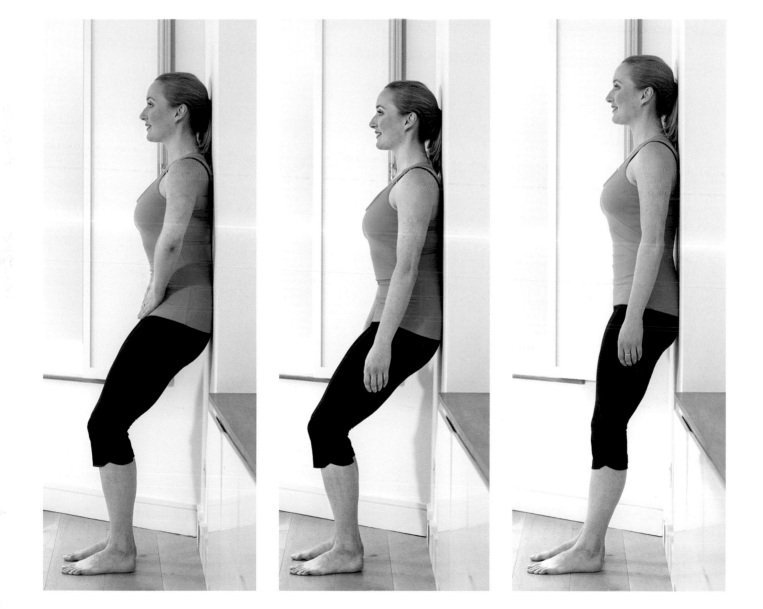

Wall Slides Variation B

Suitable for... All stages. Particularly valuable if you are Posture B, that is, if you found a reduced lumbar curve. **Aim** To develop awareness of your own individual posture and help improve your alignment.

Starting position...
Stand at a comfortable distance away from a wall – up to 30cm. Lean back into the wall. Have your feet hip-width apart and parallel. Bend your knees a little.

✳ Watchpoints

– When you have learnt how to engage your core muscles, use them to support and maintain the length of your spine.

– Be aware of the effect this movement is having on the rest of your body.

– Stay open and released across the shoulders.

– Do not tip your head back onto the wall. If it does not naturally rest on the wall allow it to balance freely on top of the spine.

– Keep your feet grounded, press the floor away evenly through both feet.

Action...

1 Place the palm of your hands into the small of your back. This should feel comfortable. Breathe in to prepare your body to move.

2 Breathe out and slowly slide down the wall a few centimetres keeping the gentle curve in your low back that your hands are helping to create. Do not allow the curve to decrease or increase.

3 Breathe in, then out as you slowly slide back up to the starting position.
Repeat *up to 8 times, after which hopefully your pelvis and spine have been encouraged to be in a mid neutral position.*
4 Now step away from the wall and keep that mid lengthened position.

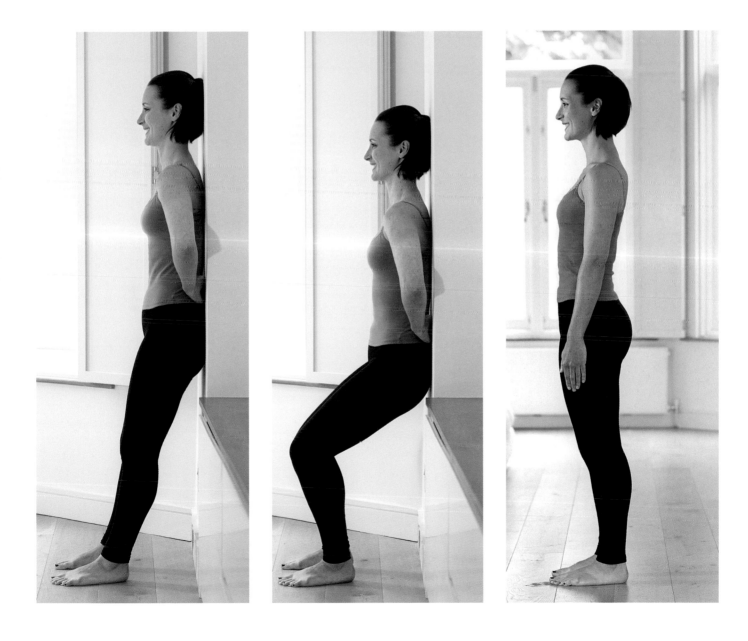

Exercise Starting Positions

We will be using lots of different starting positions in the programme; the Relaxation Position, Seated, Four-point Kneeling, High Kneeling, Prone, Side-lying and the Pilates Stance. Find which position works for you. Note that for many of the exercises they are also the position you should return to, with control, after the movement. This is as much part of the exercises as the main action!

The Relaxation Position

Suitable for... Preparing for Pregnancy, Early Pregnancy and Postnatal mothers only.

Starting position...

Lie on your back on a mat. Lengthen and release your neck, allowing the natural curves of your neck to be maintained; if necessary, place a small firm flat cushion or folded towel underneath your head. Bend your knees and place the soles of your feet firmly on the mat; your legs should be hip-width apart and parallel with one another.

Either...

✳ Place the hands on your lower abdomen with your elbows bent, resting on the mat. This arm position is suitable for relaxation and awareness.

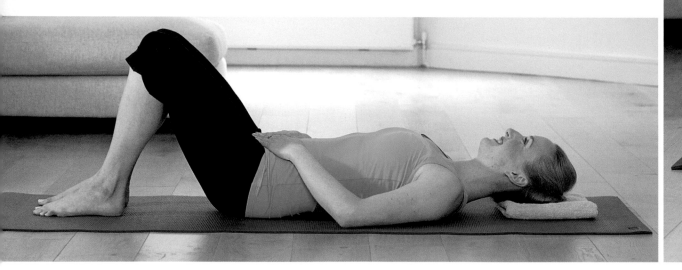

Later pregnancy option

This is not a good position to rest in but you may spend short periods in it providing you place a pillow under the right side of your trunk to tip your trunk to the left. Be alert for any signs of supine hypotensive syndrome (see page 136). This will alter your alignment, however, so is not a good position to exercise in.

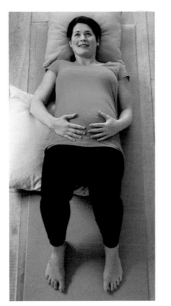

✳ Watchpoints

– Allow your entire spine to widen and lengthen as it relaxes and feels supported by the mat.

– Focus on your three areas of body weight: the back of your pelvis (sacrum); the back of your ribcage; and your head.

– Be aware of the parts of the body that are in touch with the mat and encourage them to feel heavy and supported. You will feel less contact with the mat in your lower spine. (If you are using a pillow under your hip, notice the effect this has on your pelvis and spine.)

– Release your thighs and soften the area around the hips.

– Focus on the width across your chest and feel released in the breastbone.

– Feel lengthened in your neck and release this area, as well as your jaw and the rest of your face.

– Allow time for the body to adapt to this position and allow the spine to release.

Or...

✳ Lengthen your arms by the side of your body on the mat with your palms facing down. This arm position is in preparation for movement.

The Compass

Suitable for... Preparing for Pregnancy, Early Pregnancy and Postnatal mothers only.
Aim This exercise helps develop awareness of the neutral alignment of the pelvis and lower spine. It also mobilises and releases the lower back.

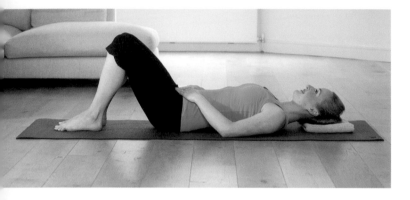

Start and finish position...

The Relaxation Position. Imagine that there is a compass on your lower abdomen; your navel is north, your pubic bone is south and the prominent bones of your pelvis on either side are west and east.

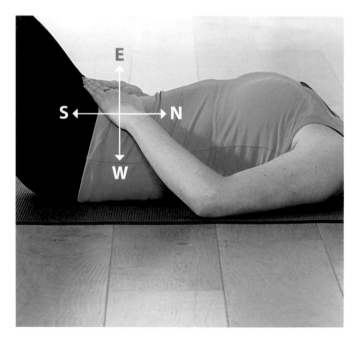

Action...

1 Breathe in, preparing your body to move.

2 Breathe out as you gently tilt your pelvis to the north (the pubic bone moves forwards and up). Feel your lower spine release into the mat as your pelvis tilts backwards.

3 Breathe in as you tilt your pelvis back through the mid-position, without stopping, until the pelvis tilts gently forwards to the south (the pubic bone moves backwards and down). Your lower back will slightly arch.

Repeat *this north / south tilt 5 times.*

4 Now, return to the Starting position and find your neutral position, which is the mid-position that is neither north nor south but in between.

5 Breathe out as you roll your pelvis to one side – east. Feel the opposite side of the pelvis lift slightly as the pelvis rotates.

6 Breathe in as you roll your pelvis through the mid-position, without stopping, to the other side – west. Feel the opposite side of your pelvis lift slightly as your pelvis rotates.

7 Return to the mid-position, the position that is neither east, west, north nor south but in between. Your pelvis is level and this is your neutral position.

- The tilt of the pelvis is very small and should feel comfortable. The rest of your spine will react slightly, but do not over-exaggerate this.
- The final neutral position should feel natural. Neutral is not a fixed or a rigid position.
- In neutral you should feel the back of the pelvis (sacrum) heavy and grounded into the mat.
- Ensure that your waist is equally lengthened on both sides.
- Also ensure that there is equal weight on both sides of the pelvis.
- Allow your hip joints to be free and released.

Quick Neutral Check

(Preparing for Pregnancy and Postnatal only) For a quick check that you are in neutral, place your hands on your lower abdomen with your hands forming a triangular shape. Your fingers touch your pubic bone and the base of your thumbs will rest approximately on your prominent pelvic bones. When you are in neutral, your fingers and thumbs are parallel to the floor and both sides of your waist are equal in length. This does not work of course when you are pregnant!

Compass in the Wall Slide Position

The Compass may also be done in a Wall Slide Position. *Suitable for...* All stages. Stand about 30cm away from a wall. Lean back into the wall. Have your feet hip-width apart and parallel. Bend your knees.

Follow the Action points opposite. Take extra care not to overarch the back going south, just move to where you are still comfortable.

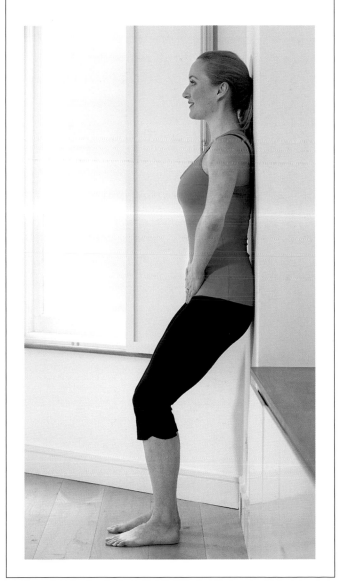

Seated Positions

You will find a variety of seated Starting positions in the book. The arm and leg positions will vary. *Suitable for...* All the Seated exercise positions are suitable for all stages.

Seated on a mat (long frog)

Take caution if you have pelvic girdle pain (see page 193).

Sit upright on the mat and position your arms and legs as follows:

✱ Bend your knees and turn your legs out from the hips and connect the soles of your feet.

✱ Your feet should be quite a distance from the body to allow a feeling of space in the hip joints. Place your hands on your shin bones; your arms are lengthened but the elbows are slightly bent.

✱ If you find it difficult to sit with a neutral pelvis and spine in this position then you can try sitting on a cushion or rolled up towel to help attain the correct alignment.

✱ You may also place pillows or cushions under your thighs for support.

Wall seated starting position

This position is useful for when you are in later pregnancy and are unable to lie flat. (Take caution if you have pelvic girdle pain.)

✱ Sit with your back to a wall. You may either sit with your legs crossed in a tailor fashion or with the soles of your feet together (Long Frog). Either way, do not have your feet too close to you as you need to allow some space around the hips. You may be more comfortable with a pillow under each knee. You may even prefer to have another pillow supporting your lower back. Take some time to make yourself feel comfortable.

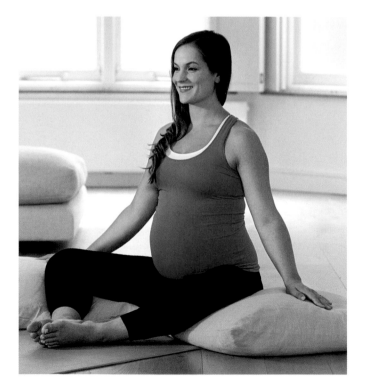
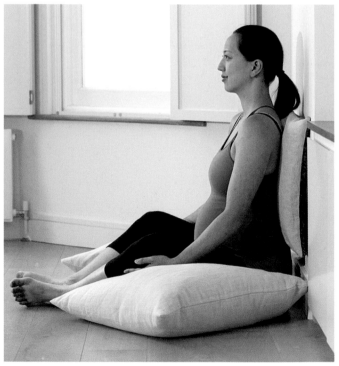

Seated on a chair

If you are going to use a chair for exercise it needs to be a sturdy upright chair.

* Sit tall on your sitting bones. You can feel these when you sit on a hard chair and place your hands under each buttock. By transferring your weight from cheek to cheek, you can feel the sitting bones. The weight should be evenly distributed between those bones.

* Have your feet planted hip-width apart either on the floor or, if you are a bit short in the leg, on a low step or pile of books.

* The back of your knee to the seat edge should be 5cm so as not to restrict blood circulation to the lower leg.

* Keep your back long with its natural 'S curve' still present.

* Supporting the lower (lumbar) back is sometimes necessary, especially if your core stabilising muscles are not yet strong enough to do the job. You may use a small cushion as support.

* Lengthen your spine and allow for the subtle, natural curvature of the lower spine

* Allow your ribcage to relax and be positioned directly above the pelvis, neither swaying backwards nor slumping forwards.

* Relax your shoulders, feel the collar-bones open and wide.

* Allow your head to balance freely on top of your spine.

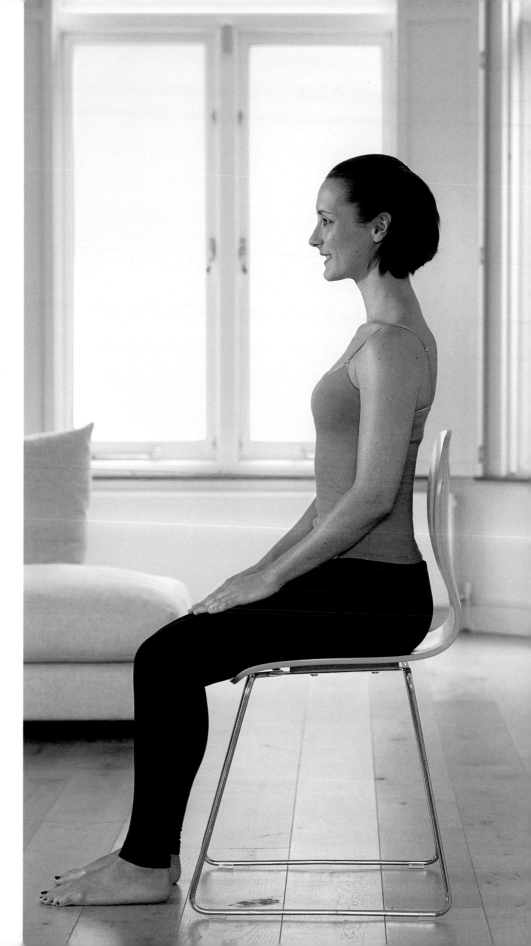

Four-point Kneeling Position

Suitable for... All stages. Take caution in the first few weeks postnatal. An incredibly useful position throughout your pregnancy, particularly towards the end. You cannot just rest in this position, you need to be active!

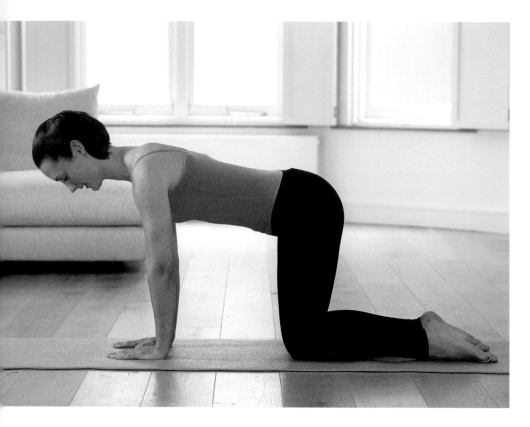

Starting position...

Kneel on all fours on the mat. Position your hands directly underneath your shoulders and your knees directly beneath your hips.

Action...

The Compass – To find the neutral position of the pelvis and lumbar spine:

1 Breathe in, preparing your body to move, and lengthen your spine.

2 Breathe out as you tilt your pelvis backwards (to north – the pubic bone moves forward) allowing your lower back to slightly round (flex).

✱ Watchpoints

– Once you have learnt how, maintain a good core connection (page 60) to avoid your pelvis and spine collapsing down towards the mat.

– The tilt of the pelvis should be small and feel comfortable. The rest of your spine will react slightly, but do not over exaggerate this.

– Fully lengthen your arms but avoid locking your elbows.

– Keep your chest and the front of your shoulders open and avoid any tension in your neck area.

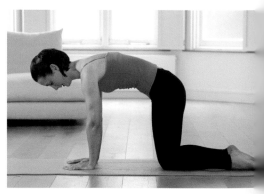

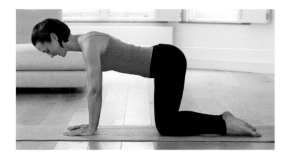

3 Breathe in and lengthen the spine and tilt the pelvis forwards (to south – the pubic bone moves backwards) allowing your lower back to slightly arch (extend).

Repeat *3 times and then find the mid-position in between these two extremes, where your pelvis is neutral (see Starting position opposite).*

This position is lengthened and level, neither tucked nor arched. Allow for the natural curvature of the lumbar spine.

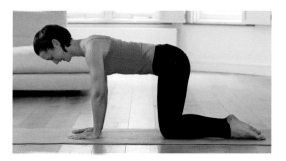

Shoulder-blade awareness – to encourage awareness of the correct position of the shoulder-blades on the ribcage.

4 Breathe in and keeping your elbows straight, gently draw your shoulder blades together (retracting them). Your chest will slightly lower towards the mat.

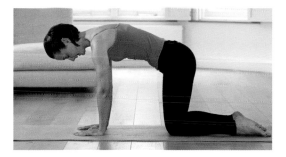

5 Breathe out as you allow your shoulder-blades to glide wider on your ribcage. Your upper spine will slightly round.

Repeat *3 times and then find the mid position of the shoulder blades in between these two extremes (see Starting position).*

Allow for the natural curvature of the upper spine and neck. Lengthen the whole spine from the crown of the head to your tailbone.

Later pregnancy option

If you find that your wrists are uncomfortable in this position, you can try placing two rolled up towels under the heel of your hands to take the pressure off the wrist.

Note that as your baby grows you will have to use your core muscles to keep the spine in good alignment.

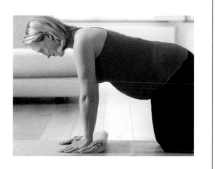

High Kneeling Position

Suitable for... All stages. Avoid if you have knee problems or simply find this position uncomfortable. High kneel on your mat. It will need to be a padded mat to protect your knees, but at the same time it should not be too padded or you will feel unstable.

✱ Your lower legs should be parallel, hip-width apart. Ensure that your weight falls not just through the knees but through the length of both shin bones evenly.

✱ Watchpoints

– Lengthen up through the spine.

– Also lengthen your waist equally on both sides.

– Allow your ribcage to relax and be positioned directly above the pelvis, neither swaying backwards, nor slumping forwards.

– Feel your shoulder-blades wide in the upper back, and your collarbones open in the front of the chest. Soften your breastbone.

– Allow your arms to hang freely in the shoulder sockets. Feel space underneath the armpits and a sense of length and weight through the hands.

– Release your neck and allow your head to balance freely on top of the spine, sense the crown of the head lengthening up to the ceiling.

– Relax your jaw muscles and focus directly forwards.

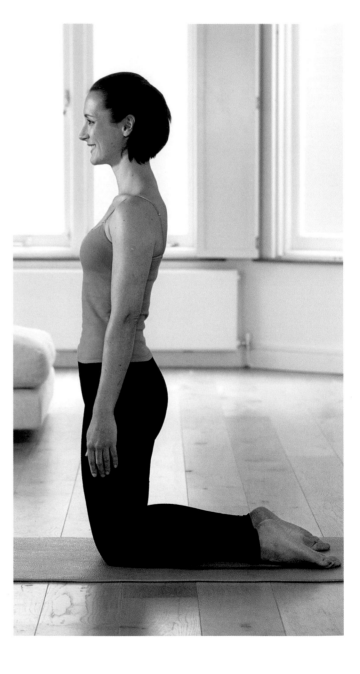

Prone Positions

Suitable for... Preparing for Pregnancy, Pregnancy up to 20 weeks and Postnatal. You will find a variety of Prone positions in the book. The arm and leg positions will vary. We have described just one version here.

If your breasts are uncomfortable in this position, you may place a flat cushion under them. Be aware, however, that this will slightly alter the alignment of your spine. You may need another flat cushion under your abdomen to avoid you dipping too much in your lower back.

* Watchpoints

* Watchpoints
–   Ensure that your weight is evenly distributed across the front of your pelvis. Avoid flattening or arching your lower spine.
–   As mentioned, if there is any discomfort in your lower spine, place a very small, flat cushion or folded towel under your abdomen. This is a temporary solution; eventually your abdominals should be strong enough to give you the support you need. Either way, your lumbar spine should feel lengthened.
–   Maintain a connection between the front of your lower ribcage and the top of your pelvis, focus on the heaviness of your ribs releasing into the mat.
–   Allow your chest to be open and although your shoulders should feel released, allow your collar-bones to widen.
–   You may place a pillow under your shins too if this helps.

*   Lie on your front in a straight line. Line yourself up in the centre of your mat to help.
*   Create a diamond shape with the arms; place the fingertips together, palms down onto the mat and open your elbows. Rest your forehead on the backs of your hands.
*   Place your legs hip-width apart and parallel.

Side-lying Positions

Suitable for... All stages. Caution if you have pelvic girdle pain (see page 193). You will find a variety of Side-lying Starting positions in the book. The head, arm and leg positions vary. We've described one version here. As your baby grows you may need several pillows for support.

Starting position...

Lie on your side in a straight line along the edge of your mat.

✻   Stretch your underneath arm away in line with your body. You will need a flat cushion between your head and arm to bring your head into line with your spine.

✻   Bend both knees in front of you so that your hips and knees are bent to a right angle. Line up hip over hip, knee over knee, shoulder over shoulder.

✻   If asked to stretch the top leg away, keep it in line with your hip as shown.

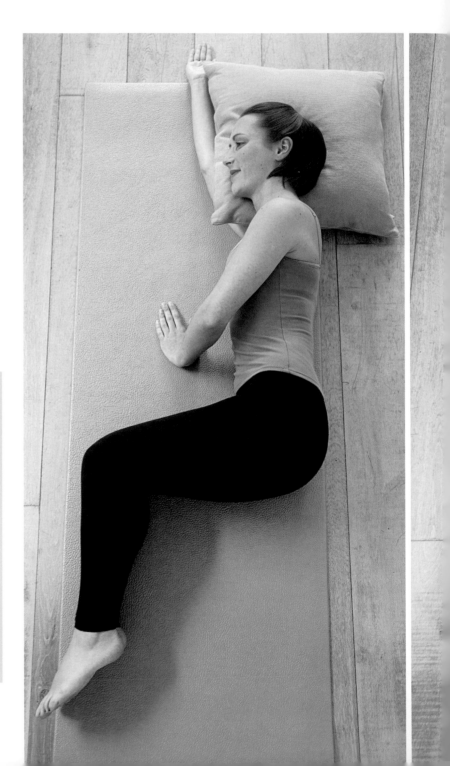

✻ Watchpoints

–   Avoid your body rolling forwards or tipping back. Imagine that you are lying in between two panes of glass and stack yourself accordingly.

–   Pelvis and spine are in neutral.

–   Lengthen both sides of your waist equally; this is essential in side-lying as it is very easy to allow the lower side of your spine to dip down towards the mat and for your spine to collapse.

–   Whether your head is supported by your outstretched arm or a cushion, ensure that it is raised sufficiently to align your head and neck with your upper spine. If your head is dropped too low or raised too high, this will affect the position and movement of the rest of your body.

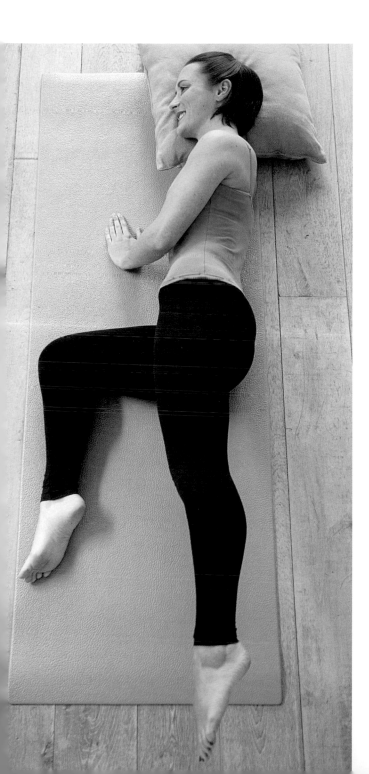

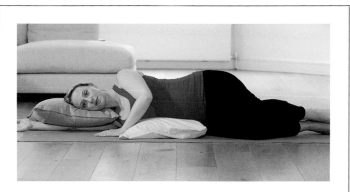

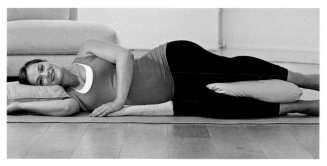

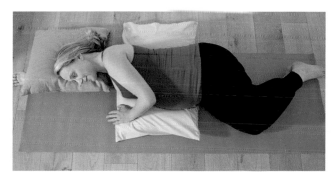

Later pregnancy options

As your pregnancy progresses you may need a few pillows or substantial cushions for support. One may be placed under your bump for support or widthways underneath your waist. Another could be placed between your knees (if they are bent).

Pilates Stance

Suitable for... All stages. Later pregnancy do not stand still for too long.

Starting position...

Stand tall on the floor (not on your mat) and slightly turn your legs out from the hips. If possible, connect your heels and place your toes slightly apart creating a small 'V position' to correspond with the turn-out in your legs.

∗ Connect your inner thighs. Allow your arms to lengthen down by the sides of your body. Transfer your weight evenly through the soles of the feet. The toes should be lengthened and without tension.

∗ Do not turn your legs out too far. Focus instead on the connection of the inner thighs, the backs of the legs and an openness in the front of the pelvis.

∗ Slightly engage the buttock muscles, drawing them up and in but avoid gripping which could lead to tightness in the lower back.

∗ Then follow the directions for Standing Alignment opposite.

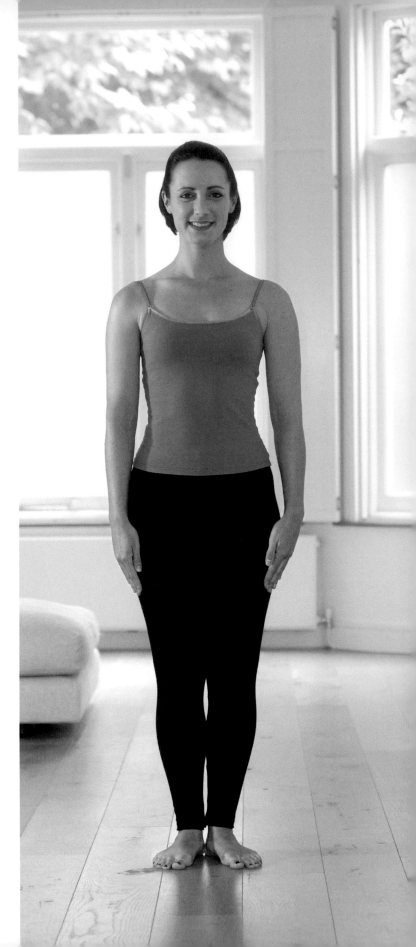

Standing Alignment

There is a tendency for most people, especially when pregnant, to carry the weight through the heels and ankles instead of over the arches of the feet. We are aiming for 80 per cent of your body weight to be balanced over the arches. This is ideal as it reduces the load on the joints created by being upright against gravity and also enables you to cope with walking on different types of surfaces. Seventeen action points to help you to stand well! This is because standing tall is an exercise rather than a 'position' – it requires you to be active.
Suitable for... All stages, but take care not to stand still for more than a few minutes while you are pregnant.

Starting position...
Stand tall on the floor (not on your mat) and place your feet hip-width apart in a natural stance, neither turned out nor in a rigid parallel position. Allow your arms to lengthen down by the sides of your body.

Action...
1 Lean forwards slightly from the ankle joint so that your weight shifts onto the balls of the feet; the heels stay down.

2 Lean backwards slightly from the ankle joint so that your weight shifts onto the heels; the toes should be lengthened and without tension.

3 Place your weight in the centre of the feet, over the arches and notice that there is a triangle of connection with the floor: a point at the base of the big toe, the little toe and the centre of the heel. The toes should be active.

4 Lengthen your legs but allow your knees to soften.

5 Tilt your pelvis forwards slightly (to south so that your pubic bone moves back and your lower back slightly arches).

6 Then passing through neutral, slightly tilt your pelvis backwards (to north so that your pubic bone moves forwards and your lower back slightly rounds).

7 Return your pelvis to your neutral position; a mid-position where the pubic bone is on the same plane as prominent pelvic bones (anterior superior iliac spines), which are also level with each other.

8 Lengthen your waist equally on both sides.

9 Find your centre by gently recruiting your pelvic floor and the deep abdominal muscles for this action (see page 60).

10 Allow your ribcage to relax and be positioned directly above the pelvis, neither swaying backwards, nor slumping forwards.

11 Feel your shoulder-blades wide in the upper back, and your collar-bones open in the front of the chest. Soften your breastbone.

12 Allow your arms to hang freely in the shoulder sockets.

Feel space underneath the armpits and a sense of length and weight through the hands.

13 Release your neck and allow your head to balance freely on top of the spine. Sense the crown of the head lengthening up to the ceiling.

14 Relax your jaw muscles and focus directly forwards.

15 While lengthening up, maintain a sense of what is happening in your lower body and be aware of the contact of your feet with the floor.

16 Breathe naturally into the ribcage.

17 This position should not feel forced or held.

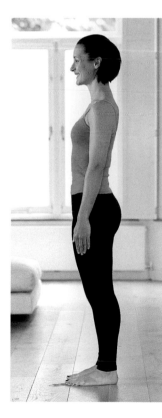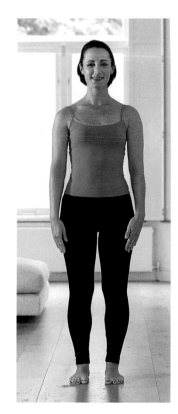

Starting position...

The Relaxation Position, lengthening your arms by your sides.

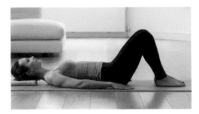

✱ Watchpoints

– The movements are very small and should feel comfortable. Be sure to perform them slowly with control.

– Maintain length in your neck, especially as you tip your head backwards.

– As you draw the chin down, ensure that the back of the head slides along the mat as opposed to simply pressing the back of the neck into the mat.

– Keep both sides of the neck long to avoid any side-bending either during the movement or in the final position.

– Try not to disturb the natural, neutral curves of your upper and lower back.

Neck Rolls and Chin Tucks

Suitable for... Preparing for Pregnancy, Early Pregnancy and Postnatal mothers. Later Pregnancy mothers may place a pillow underneath the right side of the body or try the seated version below. This exercise is designed to help you develop an awareness of neutral alignment around the head and neck. It is also a really effective way to release tension in and around the neck.

Action...

1 Breathe in, preparing your body to move.

2 Breathe out as you lengthen the back of the neck and tip your head forwards, drawing the chin down. Your neck will flex slightly; be sure to keep your head in contact with the mat.

3 Breathe in as you tip your head back gently, passing through the mid-position without stopping, to slightly extend your neck. Once again keep the back of the head in contact with the mat as the chin glides upwards; this is a small and subtle movement.

Repeat *the above 5 times and then find the mid-position where your head is neither tipped back or forwards and your neck is neither flexed nor extended. This is neutral, with your face and your focus both directed towards the ceiling.*

4 Breathe out as you keep your neck released and roll your head to one side. Again, make sure that you keep your head in contact with the mat.

5 Breathe in as you roll your head back to the centre. Repeat to the other side.

Repeat *the Neck Roll up to 5 times before returning your head back to the centre with even length on both sides of your neck.*

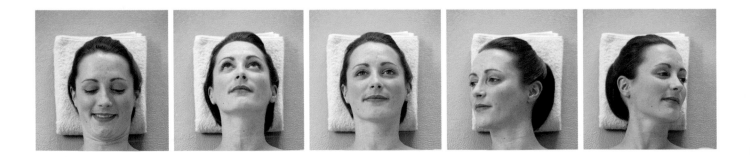

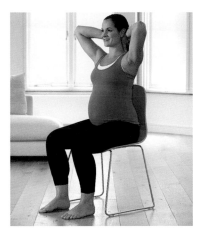

Chin Tucks (Cervical Nod)

A useful version for every stage of your pregnancy, as it helps you identify where the 'nod' comes from and how to rotate the head and neck on a central axis. Especially useful later in your pregnancy when lying flat is no longer an option. *Suitable for...* All stages.

Starting position...

Sit tall on a sturdy chair. Lightly clasp your hands behind your neck, position the hands carefully on the neck not head; in this way the neck is supported but the head can move freely.

Action...

1 Breathe in, preparing your body to move.

2 Breathe out as you lengthen the back of the neck and tip your head forwards, drawing the chin down in a nodding action. Note that your neck itself should not move.

3 Breathe in as you tip your head back gently to the start position.

Repeat *the above 5 times and then release your hands and allow your head to balance freely on top of your spine.*

* Watchpoints

– As a variation, try the cervical nod with your tongue on the roof of your mouth.

– Keep your jaw relaxed.

– Try not to disturb the natural, neutral curves of your upper and lower back.

Breathing

In the chapter on Your Changing Body we noted that breathing is an automatic process that we rarely think about. Sadly, most of us breathe far too shallowly and much faster than we need to, which may limit our oxygen supply and reduce our ability to eliminate carbon dioxide. If you use mainly only the upper part of the chest you are only using a fraction of your capacity for air. If you breathe more rapidly, you take in a new breath before emptying your lungs of the stale air. This stale air is then mixed with the fresh air decreasing your supply of oxygen and thus decreasing your energy. We want to get you breathing as efficiently as possible.

To do this we will be using different types of breathing in the programme with various end-goals in mind. While we will be using lateral thoracic breathing (Scarf Breathing) for most of the exercises, we will also be using deep abdominal breathing to encourage release of the pelvic floor (see page 108).

Remember that efficient breathing relies on good posture. It is impossible to breathe well with a hunched posture as your ribs are compressed, your thoracic cavity restricted.

We want to focus on a deeper, more rhythmic way of breathing where the diaphragm is encouraged to move up and down more which, in turn, allows the thoracic cavity to expand fully. A full inhalation followed by a deep exhalation will increase your capacity to inhale new fresh air.

We need to locate our lungs which are situated towards the back of the ribcage. To help focus on this area, try the following exercise.

Scarf Breathing
(Lateral Thoracic Breathing)

The scarf gives you sensory feedback to help you feel your ribcage expanding and closing with your breath. *Suitable for...* All stages.

Starting position...
Sit or stand tall. Wrap a stretchy scarf or stretchband around the lower part of your ribs, crossing it over at the front. Hold opposite ends of the scarf and gently pull it tight.

The inhalation...
As you breathe in, focus on the back and the sides of the ribcage where your lungs are located. Like balloons swelling gradually with air, your lungs will expand and widen the walls of your ribcage. Do not be tempted to force this inhalation as you will only create tension. You should feel the scarf tightening as your ribs expand. It is not only the filling up of the lungs that expands your ribcage but also the descent of the diaphragm, lowering into your abdominal area. Therefore your abdominal area will extend outwards. Try to breathe in through your nose and keep your shoulders relaxed.

The exhalation...
As you breathe out, feel the air gently being pushed out fully as if from the very bottom of your lungs and then exit your body via your mouth with a deep sigh. Your diaphragm will begin to rise and it will be easier to connect and hollow your deep abdominals as you consciously empty the lungs and feel the ribcage beginning to close. Do not puff your cheeks or purse your lips, as this will tense the neck, jaw and face and waste energy.

The timing...
In Pilates practice we use certain breathing patterns to help facilitate better movement. Most people find this timing difficult at first, especially if they are used to other fitness regimes. When you first practise the exercises, you may focus on controlling the movements, then, when you have those under control, you can layer on controlling your breathing. Most important of all is that you do not hold your breath or force it in any way.

Later pregnancy option

Use a seated position. When you are pregnant you are more prone to feeling dizzy, so make sure that you do not over-breathe. Your breathing should be a natural, easy pace. If you need to take an extra breath or change the timing of the breath, please do so.

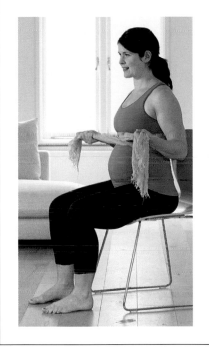

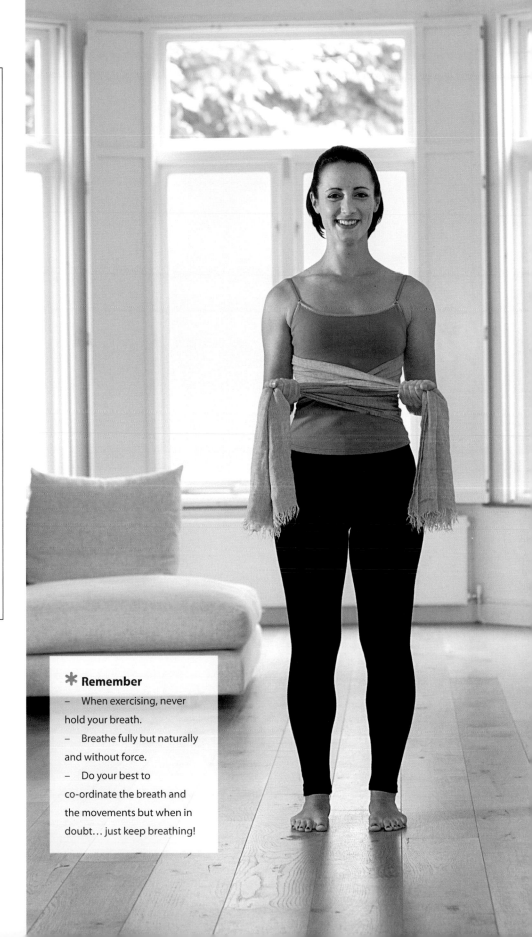

* Remember

– When exercising, never hold your breath.

– Breathe fully but naturally and without force.

– Do your best to co-ordinate the breath and the movements but when in doubt… just keep breathing!

Centring: Stability and Mobility

Centring is another of our key principles and firmly underpins the Pilates method. The term 'centring' encompasses many of the popular and widely talked about concepts associated with 'stability training'. So what do we mean here by the term 'stability'?

In general terms we would call an object stable if it can cope with the demands placed on it. For example: a stable chair is one that is built to carry the weight of the person sitting on it and can also remain upright if it is, for example, knocked. But stability can also be applied to moving objects, for example a bicycle can be stable or unstable. Or, a boat in water would be said to be stable if, when hit by a large wave, it recovers and rights itself.

When looking at our exercises, we can perhaps best view stability as being the ability to maintain control of the movements we perform. This may mean stopping unwanted movement from occurring while still allowing the desired movements to be performed.

Let's look more closely at movement itself for a moment. Movement occurs at the various joints throughout the body. Even simple movements, such as a Leg Slide (see below) involve several joints. However, if we are to keep control of the movement, some joints will have to move in a certain direction, while other joints will need to stay still.

Stability may be thought of as the process of holding still the joints that are not supposed to be moving. But it's not just about a joint staying still. The joints that are involved in the movement also need to be controlled so that they do not move before they are supposed to, or do not move in the wrong direction.

The two exercises below, Leg Slides and Spine Curls, are perfect examples of these aspects of stability. Both require a degree of pelvic and spinal stability even though the demands being placed on them are completely different movements. Leg Slides (page 62) require the pelvis and spine to remain still while the legs move. The stability of the spine and pelvis is challenged while the leg is moving.

In contrast, Spine Curls (page 72) require the pelvis and spine to move by curling them up from the mat. This demands a level of pelvic and spinal stability to stop any

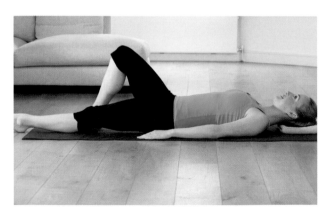

Leg Slides *See page 62*

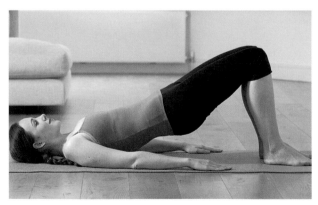

Spine Curls *See page 72*

undesired movements such as twisting or hiking up on one side.

With a clearer understanding of what we mean by stability, we can now look at 'core stability', which is what Joseph Pilates called Centring.

Core Stability is being able to stabilise and control the position of the different segments of the body, that is, the pelvis, spine, torso, shoulders and head. Think of an apple core at the heart of an apple. Gaining stability in this core area provides a stable, although not necessarily still, base of support from which all Pilates movements are initiated. To do this we have to train the core muscles. Which muscles these are will depend on what movement you are doing!

There are many different schools of Pilates, each with its own favourite way to describe how to engage your core muscles. They include cues such as 'navel to spine', 'use the powerhouse', 'stabilise', 'zip and hollow', and the list goes on. However, the words that are used are not really important, rather it's the feeling of the 'connection to inner control' that they try to convey. This connection needs to be found and used appropriately throughout each of the Pilates exercises being performed.

In this section of the book, we will focus on how to find and use this connection wisely.

Although much of the stability process is dealt with on a subconscious level, it is also possible to train and improve stability throughout the body with conscious control.

We all need stability in everyday life. However, this is never more important for you than during your ante- and postnatal periods. We have already looked at how your pregnancy hormones may make your joints prone to instability. As your baby and uterus grow your spine's stability is further challenged. Then later caring for young children inevitably requires a lot of bending, lifting, carrying, twisting. By practising Pilates, we hope to prepare your body, so that it will subconsciously react to any demand placed on it by automatically using the deep core muscles.

Pilates is based on the principle that by practising control over movements during a Pilates session, and repeating good movements, you pattern or ingrain these movements into your mind and body, thus improving the quality of your movements as you go about your daily activities.

The Dimmer Switch

When doing Pilates exercises, we encourage you to gently engage your deep stabilising muscles as necessary and keep them engaged at an appropriate level while you move. But what do we mean by 'an appropriate level'?

One of the most common mistakes made when doing 'stability training' style exercises is the over-use and over-recruitment of the core muscles. The problem is that if you engage these muscles unnecessarily or too strongly to begin with, you may end up 'fixing', becoming rigid, and thus stifling natural movement. The answer is to only engage your deep core when, and as much as you need to control the movement. No more, no less. We call this The Dimmer Switch Approach. Think of adjusting how strongly you use your core muscles as being a little like turning the dial on a dimmer switch up or down. Thus you are constantly adjusting the level to match the demands that are placed on the body.

Once you have mastered connecting to your centre with the exercises below, you can apply what you have learned to all the other exercises in this book.

Finding Your Centre: The Wind Zip (or Escalator) and Abdominal Hollowing

The focus of this exercise is simply to learn how to feel and connect to your centre. Our clients have affectionately renamed it The Wind Zip or The Escalator (travelling forward and up!) *Suitable for...* All stages (bearing in mind that when pregnant you will not achieve much of a hollow!).

To remind you to connect your centre through this zip and abdominal hollowing action during the exercises, you will see the following phrase:

Zip up to maintain a constant and appropriate connection to your centre throughout the exercise.

Starting position...

Sit upright on a chair. Place your feet on the floor, hip-width apart. Make sure that your weight is even on both sitting bones and that your spine is lengthened in neutral.

Action...

1 Breathe in to prepare and lengthen through your spine.

2 Breathe out as you gently squeeze your back passage (anus) as if trying to prevent yourself from passing wind, then bring this feeling forward towards your pubic bone as if trying to stop yourself from passing water. Continue to gently draw these pelvic floor muscles up inside. If you are not yet pregnant, you should feel your lower abdomen automatically begin to hollow.

3 Imagine you are engaging an internal zip from back to front and up inside. If pregnant, you will probably feel your bump lift gently.

4 Maintain this core connection and breathe normally for 5 breaths, you should feel that your ribs are still free to move. Then relax.

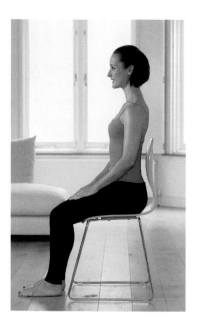

✳ Watchpoints

– Ensure that you do not zip, pull up, or pull in, too hard. It is very important that you do not force this action or grip.

– Try to keep your buttock muscles relaxed.

– Keep your chest and the front of your shoulders open and avoid any tension in your neck area.

– Keep your breathing smooth and evenly paced. Ensuring that your ribcage and abdominal area are still able to expand with your in-breath is a good sign that you haven't over-engaged.

– If you lose any of the connections, relax and start again from the beginning.

– If you find 'the zip part' too difficult, do not worry, it will come eventually.

– Try the pelvic floor exercises on pages 104–109 to help awareness of these important muscles.

– If you still find the zip too difficult focus on simply scooping the abdominals, drawing them lightly back towards the spine or, if pregnant, on gently lifting up your bump and hugging the baby from inside. At the end of the day what matters is that you are in control of your body as you move to avoid injury. This will become automatic as you practise more.

Four-point Kneeling: Connecting to your centre

We are all individuals and sometimes what works for one person may not work for another person. Trying to isolate these core muscles in a variety of positions and ways is a good idea. One will suit you best.
Suitable for... All stages. Caution in the first few weeks postnatal.

Starting position...

Four-point Kneeling. Hands directly underneath your shoulders, knees directly beneath your hips. Gently rock your pelvis and settle in the mid-position where your pelvis is neutral and the spine retains its natural curves. Lengthen the whole spine from the crown of the head to your tailbone.

Action...

1 Breathe in to prepare.

2 Breathe out as you gently squeeze your back passage (anus) as if trying to prevent yourself from passing wind, then bringing this feeling forward towards your pubic bone. Then draw these muscles up inside until you feel your abdominals automatically begin to hollow or your bump to lift.

3 Maintain this connection and breathe normally for 5 breaths before releasing, ensuring that your lower abdomen and ribs are still able to move with your breath.

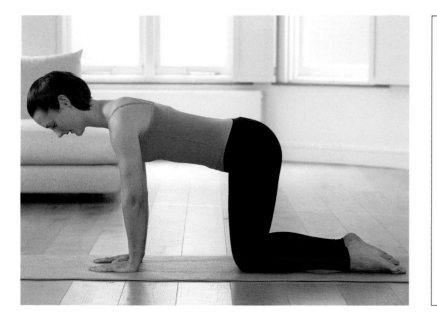

Core Variation: The 'In Between Breath' Zip

Sometimes it helps to try out an alternative breathing pattern too. In this case, you engage the core between breaths rather than on the out-breath. Breathe in and then breathe out completely, now engage the core muscles as above. Keeping the core working gently, breathe normally for five breaths before releasing. If this version works best for you, you may find it useful to engage your core this way for all the exercises in the book.

Leg Slides, Knee Openings, Single Knee Folds

Hopefully by now you are confident in how to place your body in good alignment, how to breathe laterally and how to connect to your core. Now it is time to challenge alignment while moving by trying to control your movements from a strong centre. In the following exercises, you will be learning how to move your limbs while keeping the pelvis and spine still. The Starting position for each exercise is the Relaxation Position. *Suitable for...* Preparing for Pregnancy, Early Pregnancy, Postnatal.

Leg Slides

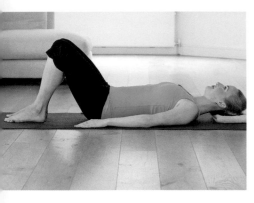 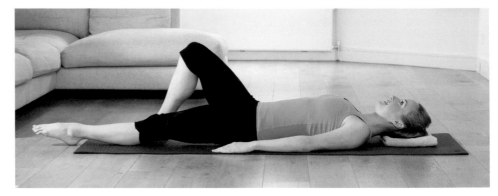

Starting position...

The Relaxation Position, arms lengthened alongside you on the mat. Or initially you may want to place your hands on your pelvis to check for unwanted movement.

Zip up to maintain a constant and appropriate connection to your centre throughout the exercise.

Action...

1 Breathe in, maintaining the connection to your centre.

2 Breathe out, as you slide one leg away along the floor in line with your hip, keeping your pelvis and spine stable and in neutral.

3 Breathe into the back of your ribcage as you return the leg to the Starting position; remain connected in your centre and keep your pelvis and spine stable and still.

Repeat *5 times with each leg.*

✱ Watchpoints

– Keep your pelvis and spine still and centred throughout.

– Focus on your waist remaining long and even on both sides as you slide your leg.

– Remain still in the supporting leg, without tension.

– Keep your foot in contact with the floor and in line with your hip.

– Keep your chest and the front of your shoulders open and avoid any tension in your neck area.

Knee Openings

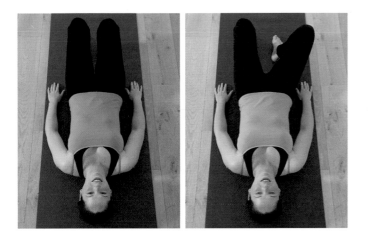

Starting position...
The Relaxation Position.

Zip up to maintain a constant and appropriate connection to your centre throughout the exercise.

Action...
1 Breathe in, preparing your body to move.

2 Breathe out as you allow one knee to slowly open to the side, keep the foot down on the mat but allow the foot to roll to the outer border. Open as far as you can without moving the pelvis.

3 Breathe in as you bring the knee back to the Starting position.

Repeat *5 times with each leg.*

> ✳ **Watchpoints** *As before plus:*
> – Focus especially on not allowing your pelvis to rock to either side.
> – Keep your supporting leg correctly aligned and still; do not allow it to open away from the working leg.

Single Knee Folds

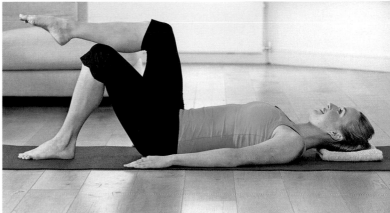

Starting position...
The Relaxation Position.

Zip up to maintain a constant and appropriate connection to your centre throughout the exercise.

Action...
1 Breathe out, as you lift your right foot off the mat and fold the knee up towards your body. Allow the weight of the leg to drop down into your hip socket and remain grounded in your pelvis and long in your spine.

2 Breathe in, maintain the position and stay centred.

3 Breathe out as you slowly return the leg down and foot to the mat.

Repeat *5 times with each leg.*

> ✳ **Watchpoints** *As before plus:*
> – Keep your pelvis and spine still and centred throughout. Focus on your leg moving in isolation to the rest of your body.
> – Fold your knee in as far as you can without disturbing the pelvis and losing neutral.
> – Fold your knee in directly in line with your hip joint.

Double Knee Folds

Suitable only for... Preparing for pregnancy. We have included Double Knee Folds here because it is a fundamental pelvic stability exercise. However, it is by no means an easy exercise to perform well and should not be attempted until you are confident with all the previous exercises in this section. A perfect demonstration of the Dimmer Switch.

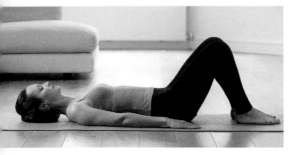

Starting position...

The Relaxation Position, arms lengthened alongside you on the mat. Or initially you may want to place your hands on your pelvis to check for unwanted movement. **Zip up to maintain a constant and appropriate connection to your centre throughout the exercise.**

Action...

1 Breathe out as you lift one foot off the mat and fold the knee up towards your body. Remain grounded in your pelvis and long in your spine.

2 Breathe in, maintain the position and stay centred.

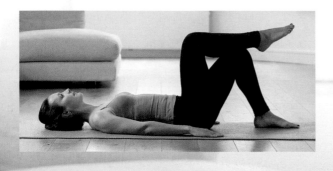

3 Breathe out as you increase your connection to your centre and fold the other knee up and towards you.

4 Breathe in, maintaining your position and staying centred as your pelvis remains grounded in neutral.

5 Breathe out as you slowly lower the foot you first folded to the mat. Do not allow the abdominals to bulge or your pelvis to lose neutral.

6 Breathe in as you slowly return the other foot to the mat.

Repeat *6 times, alternating which leg you raise and lower first.*

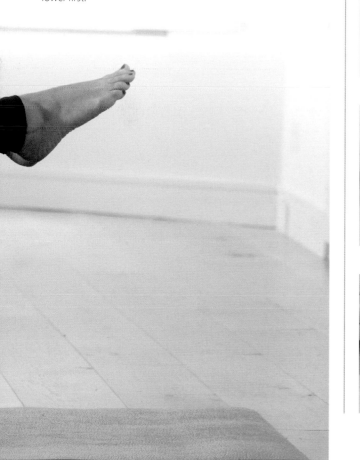

Variation

If you found this difficult, try lightly holding onto knee when it is folded in to give you extra support. Alternate which knee you support. As your core stability improves, you can lighten your hold on the knee..

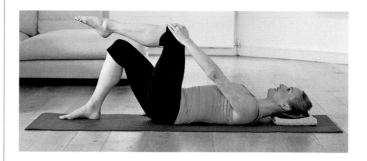

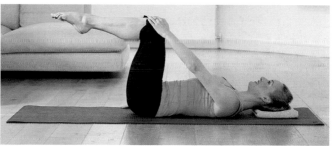

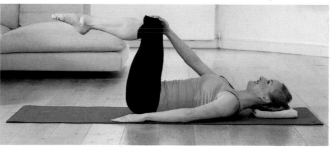

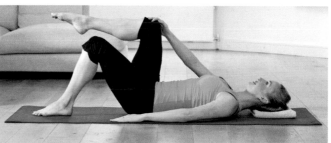

Floating Arms

We can challenge your ability to control your movements further with upper body movements. Many of us have a tendency to overuse the upper part of our shoulders which is why these muscles can get really tense. This simple exercise will help you find a way of lifting your arm that doesn't involve overuse of these muscles. As you raise your arm, think of this order of movement: first, just your arm moves up and out, then you will feel the shoulder-blade start to move – it coils down and around the back of the rib cage. Finally, the collar-bone (clavicle) will rise up. With good movement, the shoulder-blade will move in the same way as the ballast on a security barrier would move. *Suitable for...* All stages; Early and Later Pregnancy, use the seated starting position.

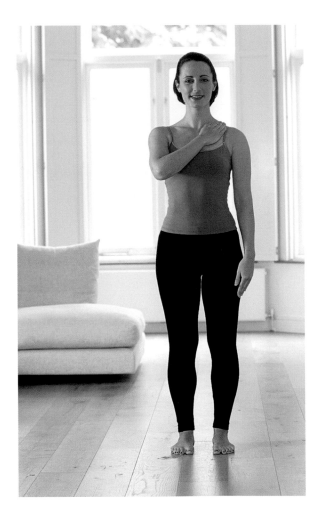

Starting position...

Stand or sit tall, remembering the instructions on page 53. Place your right hand on your left shoulder. Feel your collar bone, you are going to try to keep the collar bone still for the first part of the movement, your hand checking that the upper part of your shoulder remains 'quiet' for as long as possible. Very often this part will overwork, so think of it staying soft and released.

Zip up to maintain a constant and appropriate connection to your centre throughout the exercise.

The 'security barrier'

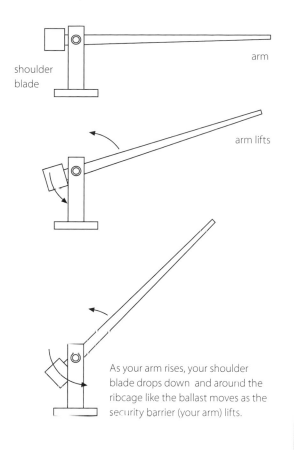

shoulder blade

arm

arm lifts

As your arm rises, your shoulder blade drops down and around the ribcage like the ballast moves as the security barrier (your arm) lifts.

Watchpoints

– Keep a sense of openness in the upper body.

– Do not allow your body to shift to the side, keep centred. Although your shoulder-blades will naturally glide upwards on the back of your ribcage as your arms rise, do not over-elevate your shoulders. It is equally as important not to depress your shoulders down your back; simply allow them to move naturally and without tension.

– Use the exhalation to encourage your breastbone to soften and close the ribcage as you raise your arms upwards.

– Without locking your elbows, keep your arms lengthened but not bent; ensure that the movement comes only from the shoulders.

Action...

1 Breathe in to prepare and lengthen up through the spine.

2 Breathe out as you slowly begin to raise the arm, reaching wide out of the shoulder-blades like a bird's wing. Think of the hand as leading the arm – the arm following the hand as it floats upwards. Keep your arm just in front of your shoulders so that it remains within peripheral vision. Allow the arm to rotate naturally within the shoulder socket as it lifts.

3 Breathe in as you lower the arm to your side, following the same pathway.
Repeat *up to 3 times with each arm.*

Ribcage Closure

With Ribcage Closure, you raise both arms simultaneously which will add further challenge to your ability to control your spine and particularly in this case your ribs! This exercise is going to be very helpful when you are pregnant as your ribcage elevates as your bump grows and doesn't always return to its pre-pregnant position after. *Suitable for...* Preparing for Pregnancy, Early Pregnancy, Postnatal. In Later Pregnancy, use Wall Slide Starting position (see opposite).

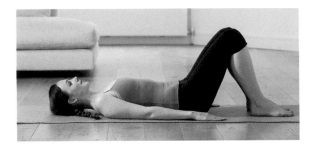

Starting position...

The Relaxation Position. Lengthen your arms by the side of your body on the mat.
Zip up to maintain a constant and appropriate connection to your centre throughout the exercise.

Action...

1 Breathe in and raise both arms to shoulder height, palms facing forwards.

2 Breathe out as you reach both arms overhead towards the floor (towards the wall if in Later Pregnancy). Keep your neck long and encourage the softening and the closing of the ribcage, keep your spine still and stable.

3 Breathe in as you return the arms above your chest. Feel your ribcage heavy and your chest open.

4 Breathe out and lower the arms, lengthening as you return them by your sides.

Repeat *up to 10 times.*

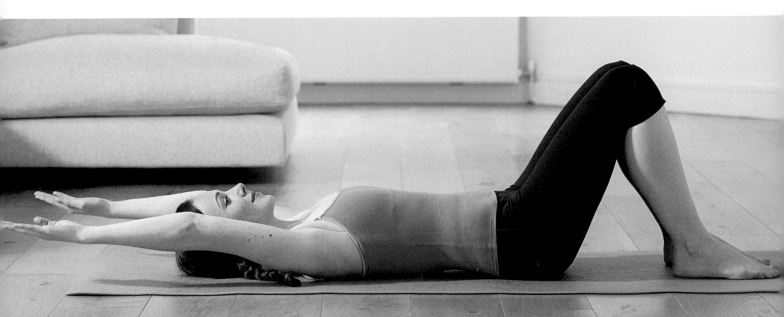

Later pregnancy option

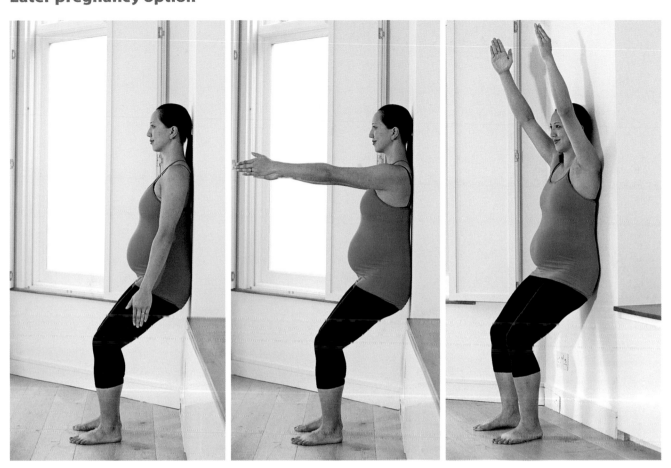

✳ Watchpoints

– Note that, unless you are very flexible, it is unlikely that your arms will reach the floor (or wall) behind you.

– Be particularly careful not to allow your upper spine to arch as you reach your arms overhead.

– Try not to over-elevate your shoulders, allow them to move naturally and without tension.

– During the exhalation, focus on the closing and softening of the ribcage.

– Fully lengthen your arms but avoid locking your elbows.

– Keep your neck long and free from tension; your head remains still and heavy throughout.

Starfish

This exercise combines everything you have learnt so far! Free flowing movement away from a strong centre. As your arm moves back think of what you learnt in Floating Arms (page 66) and Ribcage Closure (page 68). As the leg slides away think of what you learnt in Leg Slides (page 62) *Suitable for...* Preparing for Pregnancy, Early Pregnancy, Postnatal.

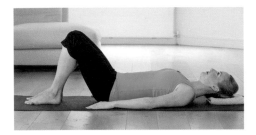

Starting position...

The Relaxation Position with your arms down by your sides.

Zip up to maintain a constant and appropriate connection to your centre throughout the exercise.

✳ Watchpoints

- As for Ribcage Closure, do not over-reach with your arms, it must feel comfortable.
- Use your core muscles to control the movement.
- The ribs stay integrated with your waist as the arm reaches away.
- Think wide and open across your collar-bones.
- Maintain the distance between your ears and your shoulders.
- The pelvis stays still and neutral when your leg slides out and when it slides back.
- Slide the leg in a line with the hip. Think of using the back of the thigh rather than the front of the thigh to bring the leg back.

Action...

1 Breathe in to prepare.

2 Breathe out as you raise one arm back as if to touch the floor behind you. You may not be able to touch the floor comfortably so only move the arm as far as you are; do not disturb the ribcage or spine. Simultaneously slide the opposite leg away along the floor in a line with your hips, keeping the pelvis stable.

3 Breathe in and enjoy lengthening away from your strong centre.

4 Breathe out and return the limbs to the Starting position.

Repeat *up to 10 times alternating arms and legs.*

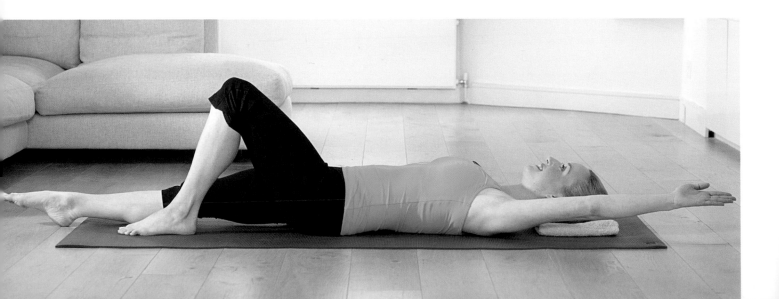

Mobility

All the exercises in Centring so far have been focused on moving the limbs independently of the pelvis, keeping your pelvis and spine still. But remember that stability is about control of movement, not about just about stillness. Remember that it's just as important for moving objects to be stable, not only still ones!

In *Return to Life through Contrology* Joseph Pilates wrote that he wanted our spines to move in a 'synchronous and smooth manner'. We are aiming for a spine that is both stable and mobile, a spine that can articulate freely, moving vertebra by vertebra in what is often referred to as segmental control. Although there is very little movement between adjacent vertebrae, it is vital to maintain this subtle movement. The total combined movement along the length of the spine allows for an almost snakelike movement.

In order to go about our normal daily activities, we need to be able to bend forwards (flexion of the spine), backwards (extension of the spine), to the side (lateral flexion of the spine) and to twist (rotation of the spine). Pilates exercises will help you learn how to control and articulate your spine segment by segment, bone by bone, through these various movements. It is important that

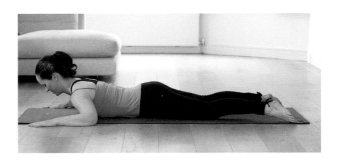

when you are planning your workouts, you should include all these movements.

A word about stretching. Normally in Pilates, we do not use passive 'stretching' (when you stay still and hold a stretch) but rather dynamic stretching, when you achieve a stretch during a movement, using one muscle group to stretch the opposing muscle group for example with Single Leg Stretch. Pilates helps improve your mobility by establishing sound movement patterns rather than simply stretching tight muscles.

It is also important to remember that we never want to force the joint beyond its range of movement. Remember this when doing your exercises; you might feel a gentle stretch but it should feel comfortable. We are going to practise just two spinal flexion exercises here.

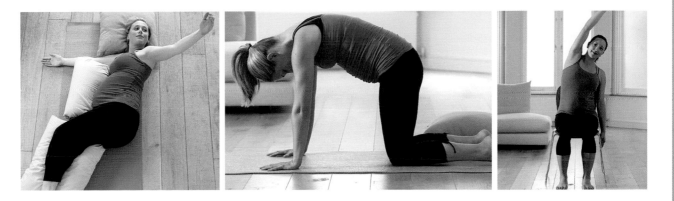

Spine Curls

The popularity of this exercise lies in its ability to gently mobilise your spine by teaching segmental control. *Suitable for...* Preparing for Pregnancy, Early Pregnancy, Postnatal.

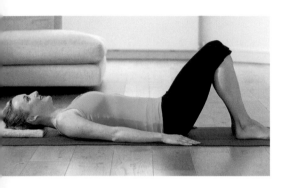

Starting position...

The Relaxation Position, arms lengthened down by the side of your body.

Zip up to maintain a constant and appropriate connection to your centre throughout the exercise.

Action...

1 Breathe in to prepare your body to move.

2 Breathe out as you curl your tailbone under, imprinting your lower back into the mat before beginning to peel your spine off the mat one vertebra at a time. Roll your spine sequentially, bone by bone to the tips of the shoulder blades.

3 Breathe in and hold this position, focusing on the length in your spine.

4 Breathe out as you roll the spine back down, softening the breastbone and wheeling once again, every single bone getting its turn.

5 Breathe in as you release the pelvis back to level again.

Repeat *up to 10 times.*

✳ Watchpoints

– Focus on wheeling your spine off the mat vertebra by vertebra on the way up and the way down.

– Avoid rolling up too far, maintain a connection of your ribs to your pelvis and avoid arching your back.

– Ensure equal weight through both feet, this will help to avoid your pelvis dipping to either side.

– Avoid 'hitching' your pelvis up towards your ribcage, keep the waist equally long on both sides.

– Keep the knees parallel, in line with your hips, and avoid your feet rolling in or out.

– Allow your collar-bones to widen and keep the neck long and free from tension.

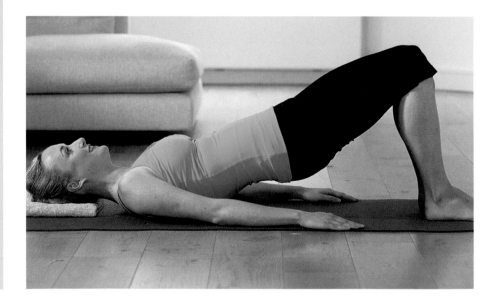

Curl Ups

Like Spine Curls this is a spinal flexion exercise but this time notice that, whereas we flexed from the bottom end in Spine Curls, in Curl Ups we flex from the top end. This exercise strengthens the abdominal muscles using them to mobilise the spine and ribcage while encouraging stability of the pelvis and legs. *Suitable for...* Preparing for Pregnancy, Early Pregnancy, Postnatal (once the abdominal divide, the diastasis recti, is 2cm or less and no bulging).

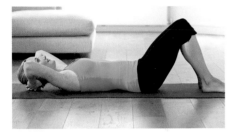

Starting position...

The Relaxation Position. Lightly clasp both hands behind your head, keeping the elbows open and positioned just in front of your ears, within your peripheral vision.
Zip up to maintain a constant and appropriate connection to your centre throughout the exercise.

Action...

1 Breathe in to prepare.

2 Breathe out as you lengthen the back of your neck and nod your head and sequentially curl up the upper body, keeping the back of your lower ribcage in contact with the mat. Keep your pelvis still and level and do not allow your abdominals to bulge.

3 Breathe in to the back of your ribcage and maintain the curled up position.

4 Breathe out as you slowly and sequentially roll the spine back down to the mat with control.

Repeat *up to 10 times.*

✳ Watchpoints

– Ensure that your pelvis remains grounded in neutral throughout; curl up only as far as this can be maintained.

– Although your pelvis remains still, allow the natural curve in your lower spine to open out and release into the mat.

– Focus on wheeling your spine off the mat vertebra by vertebra.

– Control the sequential return of your spine back down to the mat.

– Focus on your exhalation to encourage your spine to flex forwards and to close your ribcage.

– Keep a connection of the shoulder blades to the back ribcage.

– Allow your head to be heavy and supported in your hands.

– Keep the neck long and free from tension.

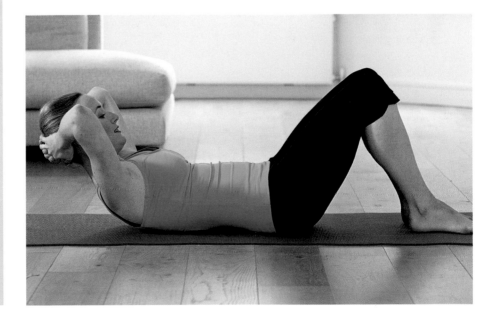

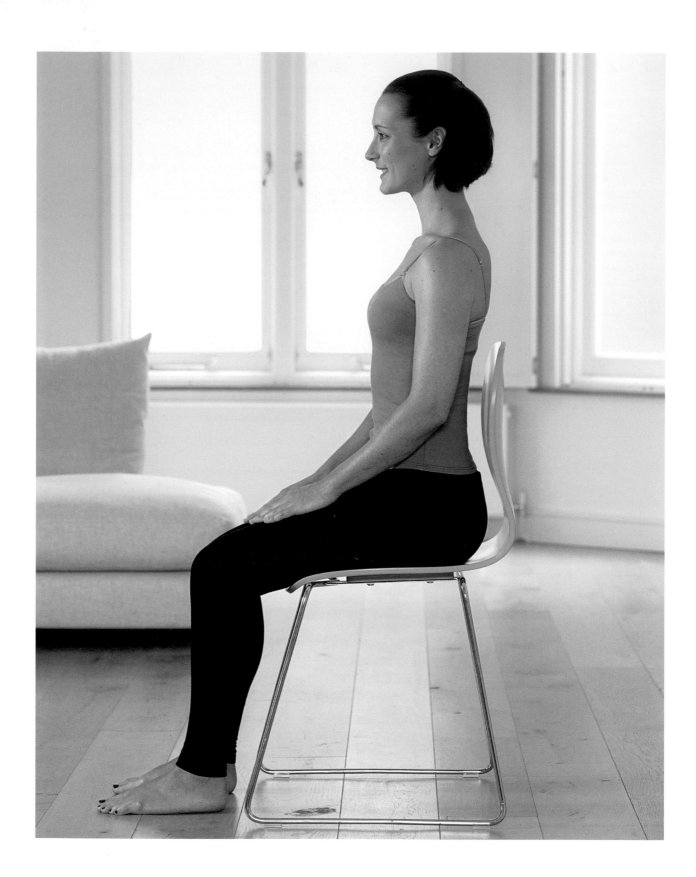

2

Preparing for Pregnancy

Preparing for Pregnancy

Not everyone has the opportunity to plan a pregnancy, but we are going to assume that as you are reading this chapter you have given yourself time to prepare for having a baby. We expect that you will use this time to organise everything in the home and at work ready for the new arrival. There's a lot to do, but may we add to the list?

It's time for you and your partner to spring-clean your bodies and get yourselves as fit and healthy as possible. Whether you are hoping for a natural conception or are undergoing fertility treatment, now is the time to make changes to your diet, exercise and general lifestyle so that you are creating the best possible environment to conceive. In this way you can help ensure a healthy pregnancy and your baby will be born into a home where wellbeing is valued. What a gift for your new child – the gift of good health.

Ideally you would allow yourself (and your partner) at least four to six months preparation time. Of course this is not always possible, nature has its own plans for conception. But this will give you time to get both your mind and your body in balance. By exercising, eating well and getting plenty of relaxation time, you can help improve both your vitality and fertility. Let's see how Pilates can help.

It's fairly obvious that anxiety and stress are not particularly conducive to baby-making activities! So learning how to relax is going to be high on our list of priorities with the exercises. Simply stopping and taking time to listen to our bodies, to be mindful and respect its needs, is something we so rarely do these days, as we juggle our busy schedules.

Taking responsibility for your own health is fundamental to Joseph Pilates's approach. As you take control, as you learn more about your body, you will find that your body confidence grows. You feel more positive about life. As you do the exercises, those feel-good hormones are released. But it is important at this time to achieve a balance. Too much exercise may be counter-productive. You will want a workout that is effective, but which does not place any unnecessary strain on the body. It is important not to do exercise that is too strenuous – you want to feel energised by your workout, not exhausted! Like anxiety and stress, add exhaustion to the list of not being conducive to baby-making! So, be sure to balance work and play, activity and rest.

One important aspect of preparing for pregnancy is to manage your weight. Research suggests that it is very important to try to be a healthy weight before you become pregnant.

But what is considered a healthy weight before pregnancy? Well, the internationally recognised way of measuring weight is to measure your body mass index (BMI). Our bodies are made up of two components: lean body mass and fat. Lean body mass consists of organs such as the heart, liver, pancreas, bones, skin and muscle tissue. All of these need oxygen and nutrients from food to grow and repair. Muscle, in particular, has a high metabolic rate and burns calories quickly. Apart from lean body mass, the rest of your body consists of fat. Fat does not need oxygen, does not repair itself and has a low metabolic rate, so it doesn't burn calories.

What we need to consider is the ratio of lean body mass to fat. This is used by doctors and fitness professionals around the world. The BMI takes into account both your height and your weight. For this, you use a set formula and you can work out your BMI using the simple equation shown in the box opposite.

Please note: your BMI is not an accurate way of measuring healthy weight DURING pregnancy or when you are breastfeeding. Only before pregnancy.

How to calculate your BMI

BMI = your weight (in kilograms) ÷ your height (in metres) squared. *For example, 60kg ÷ (1.65m x 1.65m) = 22*

1kg = 2.2lb
1m = 39in

A BMI of below 18.5 is considered underweight This means that you may need to gain weight for your health's sake. Consult your doctor if you have any concerns or if you feel afraid to put on weight.

A BMI of 18.5–25 is normal This does not mean that you cannot lose some weight for appearance's sake, but for your health you should stay in this range.

A BMI of 25–30 is overweight You should lose some weight for your health's sake.

A BMI of 30–40 is obese Your health is at risk. Losing weight will improve your health.

A BMI of over 40 is morbidly obese You should visit your doctor for a health check before you try any exercise.

If you are very overweight to the point where you would be classified as 'obese', that is if your BMI is greater than 30, then there is a greater risk of your baby becoming obese in later life. The National Institute for Health and Clinical Excellence published a report in 2010 advising that 'women should be encouraged to achieve a healthy weight before they become pregnant, and advised that 'there is no need to "eat for two" when pregnant'. The guidelines advise that women who have a BMI of 30 or more should be advised that even losing lose 5–10 per cent of their weight would have significant health benefits and could increase their chances of becoming pregnant.

Dieting during pregnancy is not recommended as it may harm the health of the unborn child which is why it makes good sense to get your weight under control before you become pregnant. This is best done by following a healthy balanced diet and increasing your levels of activity. It is fine to exercise to help you lose weight before you become pregnant, but remember that over-exercising is not going to help!

Being underweight can also affect your ability to conceive. We all need some body fat. If you have too little body fat, you may run the risk of decreased fertility associated with amenorrhoea (when menstruation ceases). Practising Pilates is a great way to manage your weight and keep this balance. It is not so strenuous that you risk overdoing it but it will help you build muscle and thus improve your ratio of lean body mass to fat.

How else can Pilates help you prepare for pregnancy?

The exercises work on improving your posture and breathing. We have already seen in the chapter on Your Changing Body, how poor posture can affect health. It may interrupt the flow of blood and thus its ability to distribute the oxygen and nutrients needed for repair and growth. It may also affect its capacity to remove toxins from your system. If we are going to spring-clean your body, we want everything to be working efficiently. We are also going to prepare your abdominal muscles for the role ahead. We noted before that when you are pregnant your abdominals are going to have to stretch to accommodate the growing baby. While this is inevitable, there is lots we can do to ensure that your 'natural corset' of muscles continues to support your back and the growing weight of the baby. Good core muscles should help prevent the abdominal divide (diastasis recti) from being a lasting problem. However, once again we have to look for the right balance. We are looking for abdominal muscles that are sufficiently strong but also flexible. To do this we can match exercises, like Curl Ups, which strengthen your abdominals, with exercises such as Dart and Star, which help to lengthen out your abdominals. But we will not be including some of the more challenging Pilates exercises. We do not want to overwork or overstretch your abdominals at a time when you may become pregnant.

Which brings us to that moment when you first suspect that you may be pregnant. As we mentioned in 'How to use this book', may we ask you not to exercise until you have spoken to your doctor? Hopefully, your doctor will give you permission to continue to exercise, but may advise you to wait until you are 16 weeks or even to wait until you have given birth. Only your doctor has your full medical history.

If you have a normal pregnancy with no complications and if you have been doing regular Pilates over the past 4–6 months, then hopefully you can exercise through your first trimester. In which case please turn to page 110 for the Early Pregnancy Programme.

If your doctor advises you to wait, you can always rejoin the programme at 16 weeks (or whenever they advise) with the Later Pregnancy exercises.

By following The Fundamentals and this Preparing for Pregnancy programme, you will have already laid the best possible foundations for good Pilates practice.

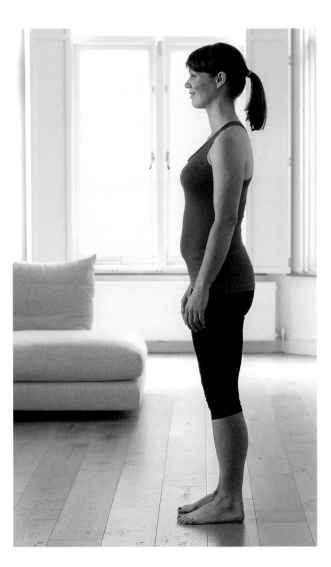

Preparing for Pregnancy Workouts

We can summarise the goal of this section in one word: Balance! In addition to the exercises in this chapter you can also choose any exercise from the rest of the book. The workouts given below will help you achieve just that and ideally you and your partner will practise together.

When creating your own workouts, try to include exercises for all the spinal movements, flexion, rotation, side flexion and extension. Try also to balance upper and lower body work.

We have given you below two sample workouts: one using exercises from The Fundamentals and Preparing for Pregnancy: the second workout also using exercises from the rest of the book.

Workout One

Shoulder Drop Variation . . . . (page 81)

Neck Rolls . . . . (page 54)

Pillow Squeeze . . . . (page 106)

Starfish . . . . (page 70)

Knee Circles . . . . (page 120)

Pelvic Clocks . . . . (page 92)

Curl up with Knee Opening . . . . (page 84)

Spine Curl with Ribcage Closure . . . . (page 82)

Oblique Curls . . . . (page 86)

Hip Rolls . . . . (page 93)

Single Leg Stretch . . . . (page 71)

Arm Openings . . . . (page 160)

Dart . . . . (page 94)

Star . . . . (page 95)

Table Top . . . . (page 96)

Rest Position . . . . (page 98)

Side Reach (standing) . . . . (page 100)

Tennis Ball Rising . . . . (page 127)

Roll Downs . . . . (page 102)

Workout Two

Wall Slides A or B . . . . (pages 36–39)

Ribcage Closure (in Wall Slide) . . . . (page 69)

Nose Spirals . . . . (page 117)

Spine Curls with Knee Opening . . . . (page 201)

Curl Ups with Leg Extension . . . . (page 121)

Knee Rolls . . . . (page 116)

Oblique Curls with Leg Slide . . . . (page 87)

Oyster . . . . (page 161)

Side-lying Circles . . . . (page 166)

Star Variation . . . . (page 123)

Crawling Lizard . . . . (page 208)

Oblique Cat . . . . (page 125)

Side Reach (seated on mat) . . . . (page 100)

Pelvic Floor Control exercises . . . . (pages 104–109)

Waist Twist (standing) . . . . (page 127)

Dumb Waiter . . . . (page 157)

Pilates Stance . . . . (page 52)

Chest Expansion . . . . (page 154)

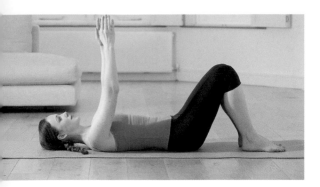

Shoulder Drops and Variations

This one is magic, like giving yourself a shoulder massage. It also teaches you good alignment of the shoulders. *Suitable for...* Preparing for Pregnancy, Early Pregnancy, Postnatal.

Starting position...

The Relaxation Position. Raise both arms vertically above your chest, shoulder-width apart, with your palms facing one another.
Zip up to maintain a constant and appropriate connection to your centre throughout the exercise.

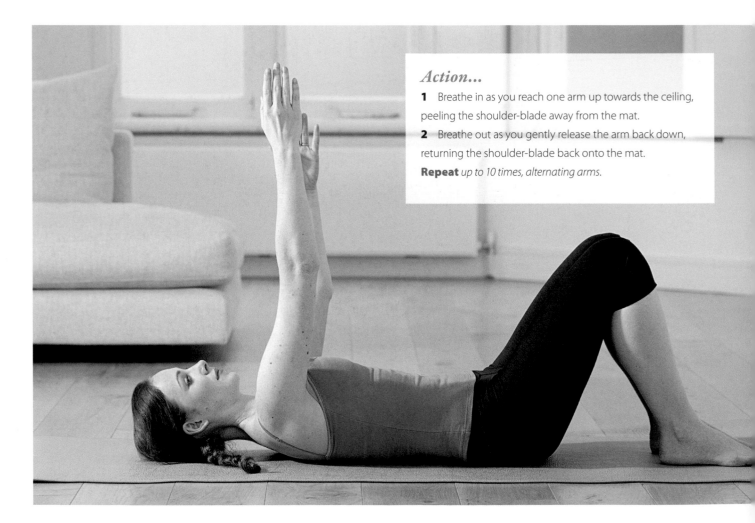

Action...

1 Breathe in as you reach one arm up towards the ceiling, peeling the shoulder-blade away from the mat.
2 Breathe out as you gently release the arm back down, returning the shoulder-blade back onto the mat.
Repeat *up to 10 times, alternating arms.*

Later pregnancy option

Try Seated by a wall or Seated on a chair as a Starting position. Unfortunately you miss the pull of gravity to help release the shoulders but if you have a stretch band, you can wrap this around your chest just under your shoulder-blades. Follow the directions below and you'll find that the retraction of the band mimics the pull of gravity.

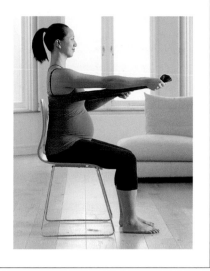

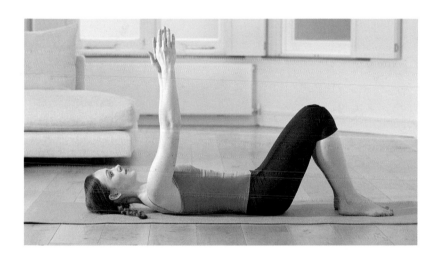

Variation 1

Reach and release both arms at the same time.

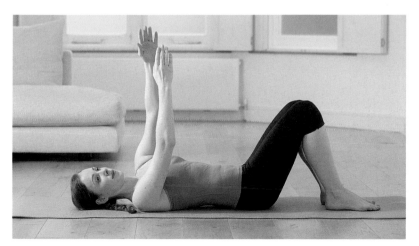

Variation 2

Follow the direction above but reach across your body to achieve an extra stretch between the shoulder-blades. Try to keep the pelvis central as you reach.

Spine Curls with Ribcage Closure

A firm favourite with everyone. This is the ultimate feel-good exercise. Gently mobilises your spine and hips while strengthening your back muscles, abdominals, buttocks and hamstrings (back of your legs). Just take a minute to revise Ribcage Closure on page 68. *Suitable for...* Preparing for Pregnancy, Early Pregnancy, Postnatal.

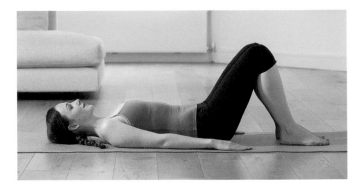

Starting position...

The Relaxation Position, arms lengthened down by the side of your body.

Zip up to maintain a constant and appropriate connection to your centre throughout the exercise.

Action...

1 Breathe in to prepare your body to move.

2 Breathe out as you curl your tailbone under, imprinting your lower back into the mat before beginning to peel your spine off the mat one vertebra at a time. Roll your spine sequentially, bone by bone to the tips of the shoulder-blades.

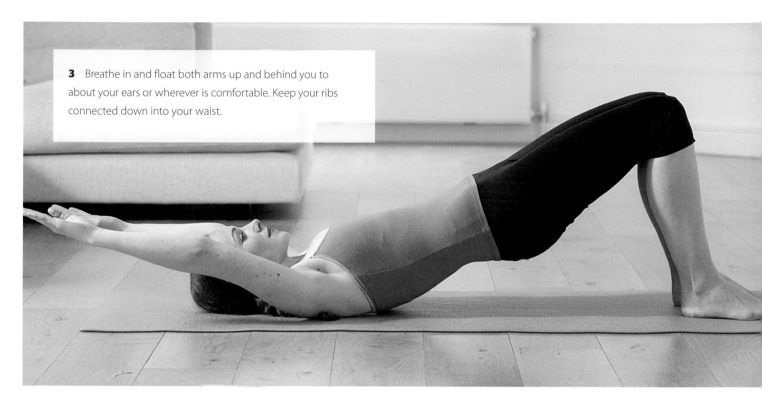

3 Breathe in and float both arms up and behind you to about your ears or wherever is comfortable. Keep your ribs connected down into your waist.

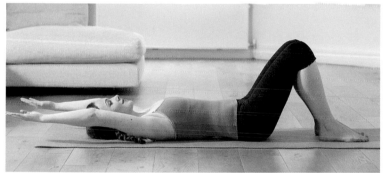

4 Breathe out as you roll the spine back down, softening the breastbone and wheeling once again, every single bone getting its turn.

5 Breathe in as you bring your arms back to the Starting position and release the pelvis back to level again.

Repeat *up to 10 times.*

---

* **Watchpoints**

- Focus on wheeling vertebra by vertebra.
- Avoid rolling up too far; maintain a connection of your ribs to your pelvis and avoid arching your spine especially as your arms reach back.
- Do not force your arms onto the floor behind you.
- Ensure equal weight through both feet; this will help to avoid your pelvis dipping to either side.
- Try to avoid 'hitching' your pelvis up towards your ribcage, keep the waist equally long on both sides.
- Keep the knees parallel, in line with your hips, and avoid your feet rolling in or out.
- Maintain length through the back of the neck, particularly avoiding your head tipping back as your spine rolls down.

Curl Ups with Knee Openings

Normally we would promote this exercise as perfect for achieving a flat stomach. It is, but bearing in mind the long-term goal here, we can settle for it improving your core stability! For good measure, we also added an extra element (the Knee Opening) to challenge your pelvic stability. *Suitable for...* Preparing for Pregnancy, Early Pregnancy and Postnatal (once the diastasis recti is less than 2cm). If you had a caesarean section, wait 5 months.

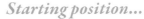

Starting position...

The Relaxation Position. Lightly clasp both hands behind your head, keeping the elbows open and positioned just in front of your ears, within your peripheral vision.

Zip up to maintain a constant and appropriate connection to your centre throughout the exercise.

1   Breathe in, preparing your body to move.

2   Breathe out as you lengthen the back of your neck, nod your head and sequentially curl up the upper body, keeping the back of your lower ribcage in contact with the mat. Keep your pelvis still and level and do not allow your abdominals to bulge.

3 Breathe into the back of your ribcage and maintain the curled up position.

4 Breathe out as you slowly open one knee to the side, keeping your pelvis still and stable.

5 Breathe in as you bring the knee back in line with the hip.

✳ Watchpoints

– Focus on wheeling your spine off the mat vertebra by vertebra and remember that curling back down sequentially is just as important.

– Allow your head to be heavy and supported in your hands, allowing your neck to be free from tension.

– As the knee opens to the side, allow the foot to roll onto the outside edge.

– As the knee draws back into line again with the hip, the foot rolls back and centres.

– Only move the leg to the side as far as you can without disturbing the pelvis.

– As you breathe in, breathe into the back of the ribs to help you stay curled up.

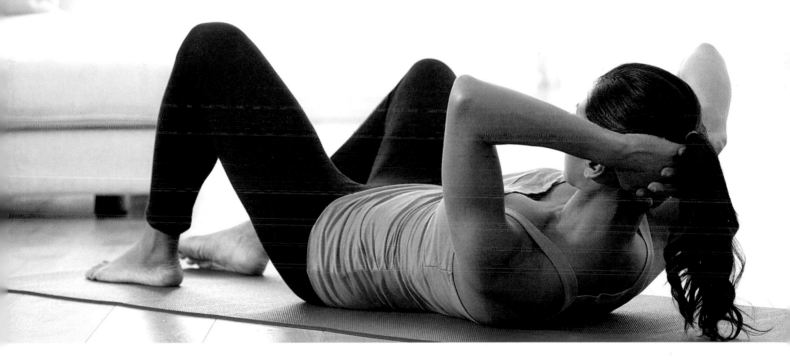

6 Breathe out and open the other knee with control.

7 Breathe in as you bring this knee back in line.

8 Breathe out as you roll the spine back down to the mat.
Repeat *up to 5 times*.

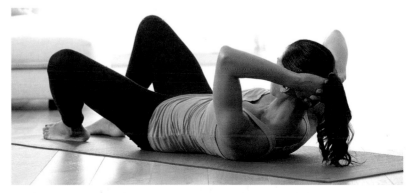

Oblique Curl Ups

Like Curl Ups, this exercise strengthens the abdominal muscles, using them to mobilise the spine and ribcage. The addition of rotation to the curling movement adds another dimension of challenge to the exercise, particularly when it comes to maintaining the stability of the pelvis and legs. *Suitable for...* Preparing for Pregnancy, Early Pregnancy, Postnatal (once the diastasis has improved and is less than 2cm). Wait at least 8 weeks before adding this exercise to your programme as it requires stronger abdominal muscles than Curl Ups. If you have had a caesarean section, wait 5 months.

Starting position...

The Relaxation Position. Lightly clasp both hands behind your head, keeping the elbows open and positioned just in front of your ears, within your peripheral vision. **Zip up to maintain a constant and appropriate connection to your centre throughout the exercise.**

✳ Watchpoints *As for Curl Ups plus:*

– Ensure that your pelvis remains grounded, central and in neutral throughout. Curl up only as far as this can be maintained.

– The rotation should come from the movement of the ribs on the spine and the spine itself. Try not to pull on your head and neck.

– Keep both sides of the waist equally long.

– Maintain openness across your back, shoulders and chest by directing your elbows wide and forwards

– Allow your head to be heavy and supported in your hands. Rotate your head in relation to the rotation in your spine; no more and no less.

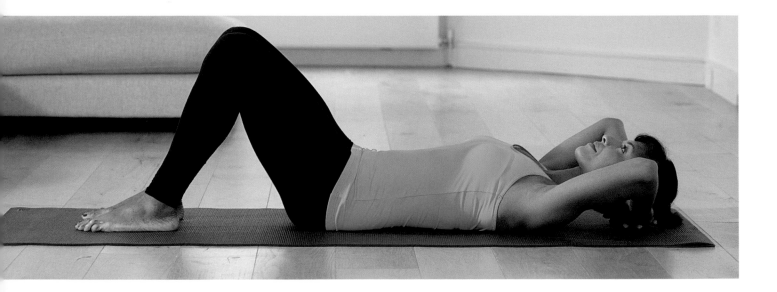

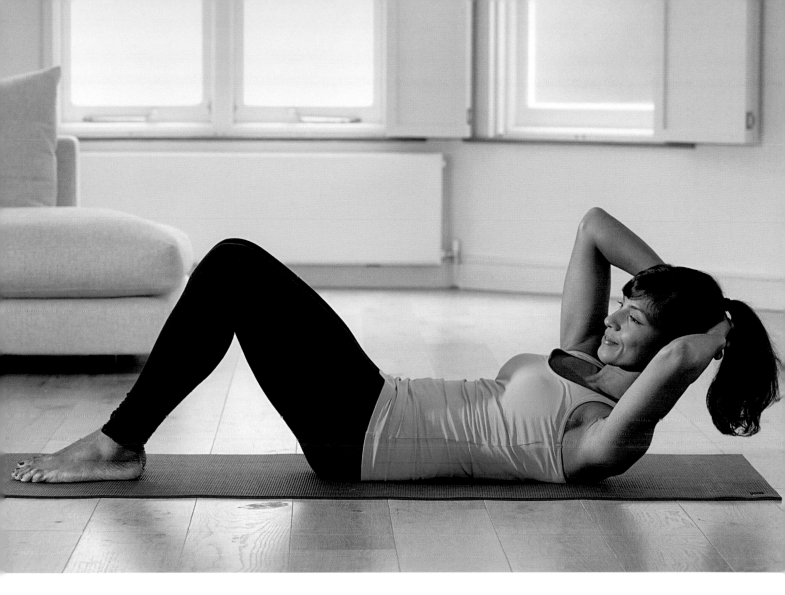

Action...

1 Breathe in to prepare your body to move.

2 Breathe out as you nod your head and sequentially curl up the upper body, rotating your head and torso to the left and directing the right side of your ribcage towards your left hip. Keep your pelvis still and level and do not allow your abdominals to bulge.

3 Breathe in to the back of your ribcage and maintain the curled and rotated position.

4 Breathe out as you slowly and sequentially roll back down to the centre with control.

5 Repeat, this time rotating to the right.

Repeat *up to 10 times.*

Variation

Oblique Curl Ups with Opposite Leg Slide

As above but as you curl up, lengthen the opposite leg away in a Leg Slide action. Stay aware of moving around your centre axis.

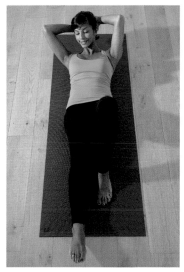

Single Leg Stretch Stage 1

We are going to learn this classical exercise in stages of increasing difficulty. Do not overstretch and make sure that you are very comfortable with one stage before moving onto the next. This first stage is to familiarise yourself with the arm movement, co-ordinating it with your breath. Once you are pregnant, your hormones will affect your hand to eye co-ordination and spatial awareness so this may prove a worthy challenge. *Suitable for...* All stages.

Starting position...

Sit tall on the edge of your mat with your knees bent in front of you. You may sit on a rolled up towel if this helps. Place your hands onto the outside of your shinbones.
Zip up to maintain a constant and appropriate connection to your centre throughout the exercise.

Action...

1 Breathe into the back of your ribcage.

2 Breathe out as you slide your right leg forwards in line with the hip. Simultaneously place the right hand on the left knee.

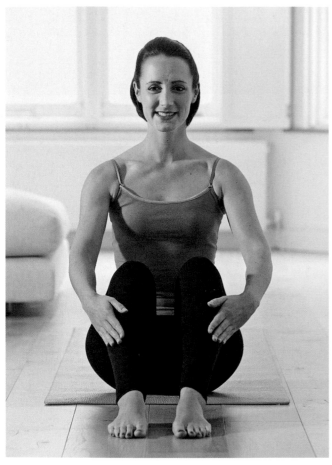
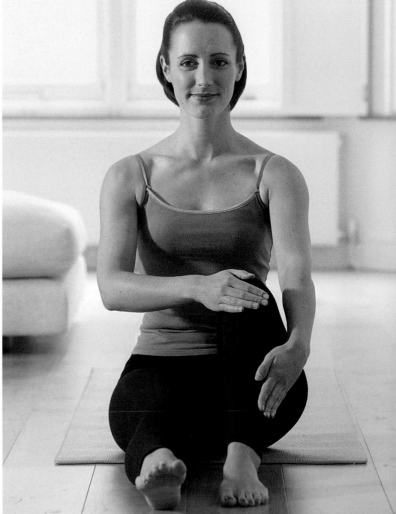

3 Continue to breathe out as you switch legs, bending the right leg in and stretching the left leg away. Your left hand will now be positioned on the right knee and the right hand on the right shin bone.

4 Breathe in as you repeat a further two leg stretches, firstly stretching your right leg away and then your left leg.

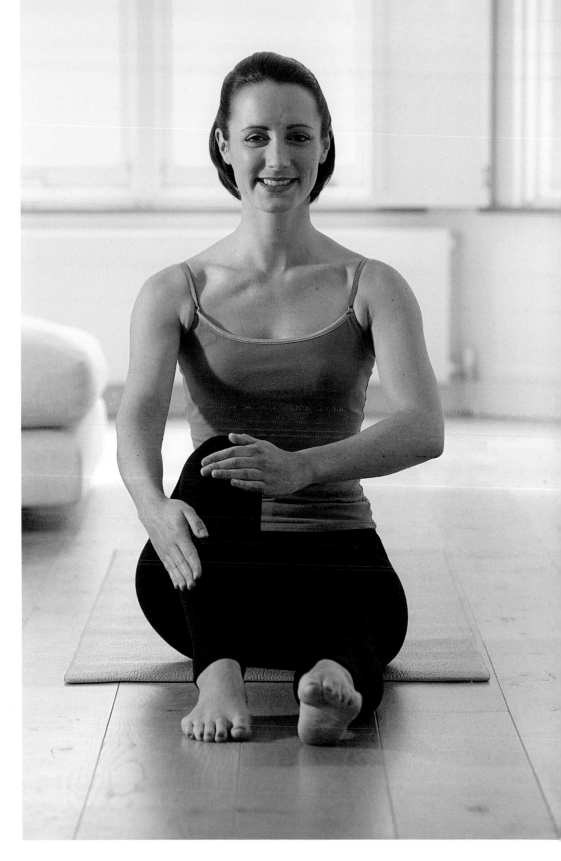

✱ Watchpoints
- Keep your upper body open, elbows soft, neck and chest muscles released.
- Keep lifting up out of your waist which should stay equally lengthened on both sides.
- Check that your weight stays even on both sitting bones.

Single Leg Stretch Stage 1

This is the most challenging abdominal exercise in the book. It brings together all the skills you have learnt so far. *Suitable for...* Preparing for Pregnancy, Postnatal only after 3 months when you feel completely back to normal and there is no doming at all. Revise Curl Ups (page 72) and Double Knee Folds (page 64) first.

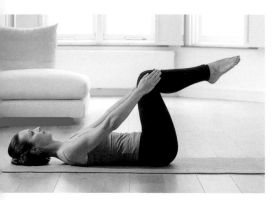

Starting position...

The Relaxation Position. Double Knee Fold one leg at a time with stability. Place your hands onto the outside of your shin-bones. The legs are slightly turned out from the hips, the heels are connected and the knees hip-width apart.
Zip up to maintain a constant and appropriate connection to your centre throughout the exercise.

Action...

1 Breathe into the back of your ribcage.
2 Breathe out as you nod the head and curl up.

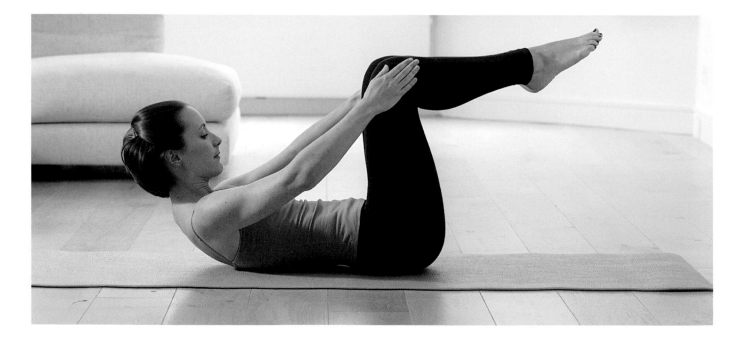

3 Breathe into the back of the ribcage to stay curled up.

4 Breathe out as you stretch and press your right leg forwards in line with the hip at an angle of about 45° above the mat. Simultaneously place the right hand on the left knee.

5 Breathe in and bend the right leg back in, returning the right hand to the shin-bone.

6 Breathe out as you stretch the left leg away, placing the left hand on the right knee.

7 Breathe in and bend the left knee back in, returning the left hand to the left shin-bone.

Repeat *up to 8 times, before lowering the feet one at a time and slowly curling back down with control.*

✱ **Watchpoints**

–   Keep the back anchored, pelvis square and the sacrum centred on the mat, if necessary extend the leg higher into the air.

–   Move the legs smoothly with control from the hip joints, keeping in line with the hip joints.

–   Softly point the feet throughout.

–   Both sides of the waist remain equally lengthened.

–   Turn your core connection up or down as appropriate to control the movement and keep your back anchored.

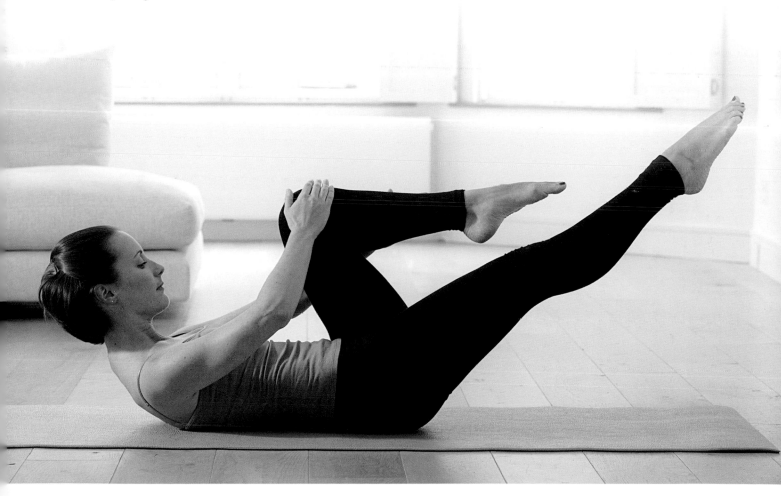

Pelvic Clocks

A fun exercise, which helps to bring blood flow to this area, develop awareness of the position of your pelvis and mobilise and release the hips and lumbar spine. While labour may seem a long way off, Pelvic Clocks may be helpful for managing your contractions during labour. *Suitable for...* Preparing for Pregnancy, Early Pregnancy, Postnatal. Later Pregnancy mothers should use an alternative Starting position such as Four-point Kneeling, High Kneeling, Standing (knees slightly bent).

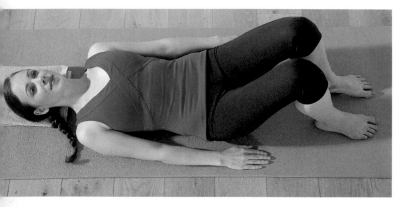

Starting position...

The Relaxation Position. Imagine that there is a clock face on the lower abdomen; the navel is 12 o'clock, the pubic bone 6 o'clock, the most prominent front part of your pelvic bones are 3 o'clock and 9 o'clock on either side. Visualise a marble in the middle of the clock face.

Zip up to maintain a constant and appropriate connection to your centre throughout the exercise.

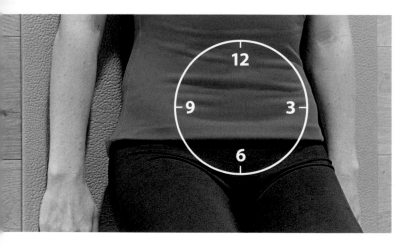

Action...

1   Breathe in to prepare the body.

2   Breathe out and tilt your pelvis back as you visualise the marble rolling to 12 o'clock.

3   Breathe in there, and as you breathe out continue to roll the marble around to 1 o'clock and so on, rotating the pelvis until arriving at 6 o'clock where the pelvis will be centred and tilted forward. If you know that you have an increased lumbar lordosis (Posture A), take care not to over-arch your back at this point.

4   Breathe in and start to roll the marble around up to 7 o'clock and so on, rotating the pelvis until arriving in the centre once again in a posterior tilt at 12 o'clock.

Repeat *up to 5 times and then repeat 5 times in the opposite direction before settling back into a neutral position. Take an extra breath on the way round to 12 o'clock if you need to..*

Variation

If you find this breathing pattern too complex, simply breathe normally throughout the exercise.

✳ Watchpoints

–   Enjoy the free movement of your pelvis but stay in control. Think belly dancer!

–   Keep both sides of your waist equally lengthened.

–   Try to keep your knees still.

Hip Rolls

This is a great rotation exercise. It is very easy just to allow the weight of the legs to pull you over. The skill is to use appropriate core control to roll sequentially. Works the obliques and thus is great for the waistline. *Suitable for...* All stages. Later Pregnancy: note that you are moving, so it is fine for you but do not rest in the Relaxation Position and remain alert for any signs of supine hypotensive syndrome (page 136).

Starting position...

The Relaxation Position. Bring your legs together and connect your inner thighs. Reach your arms out on the mat slightly lower than shoulder height with your palms facing upwards.
Zip up to maintain a constant and appropriate connection to your centre throughout the exercise.

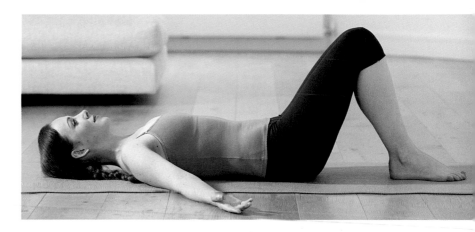

Action...

1 Breathe in to prepare.
2 Breathe out and maintaining the connection of the inner thighs, begin to rotate your pelvis and legs to the right. The left side of the pelvis and the lower left ribs will peel slightly off the mat.
3 Breathe in and hold the position.
4 Breathe out as you return the pelvis and legs back to the Starting position initiating the roll from your centre.
Repeat *on the other side and then repeat the whole sequence up to 5 times.*

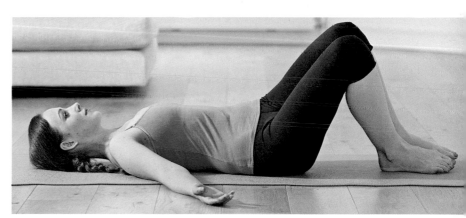

✳ Watchpoints
- Roll your pelvis and your legs directly to the side, there should be no shortening on either side of the waist.
- Maintain a connection between your ribcage and your pelvis and ensure that you don't arch your back as you roll.
- Control the movement of your legs and don't just allow them to 'drop' to the side.
- Ensure the foot on top peels away from the mat during the roll.
- Keep your chest and the front of your shoulders open and avoid any tension in your neck area.

Dart

An important exercise for correcting poor posture and strengthening the back muscles. *Suitable for...* Preparing for Pregnancy, Pregnancy up to 20 weeks (but avoid if you feel uncomfortable), Postnatal. **Equipment** Folded towel (for forehead), small flat cushion (optional).

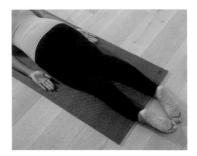

Starting position...

Lie on your front in a straight line. Rest your forehead on a folded towel. Lengthen your arms by the side of your body, palms facing the ceiling. Your legs are straight but relaxed, the base of your big toes touching. You may place a flat cushion underneath your abdomen to support your lower back. Before we begin, take a look at the leg action in the photos on the left.

Zip up to maintain a constant and appropriate connection to your centre throughout the exercise.

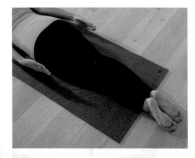

Action...

1 Breathe in to prepare.

2 Breathe out as you lift first your head, then your neck and then your chest and upper spine off the mat. Feel your lower ribs remaining in contact with the mat. Lengthen your arms away and lift them slightly as they turn in, palms facing your body. Simultaneously draw your legs together connecting the inner thighs in a parallel position.

3 Breathe in as you hold this lengthened and stable position, feeling the opposition of the crown of your head reaching away from your toes.

4 Breathe out as you return the spine and head sequentially back down to the mat, with control, simultaneously releasing your legs and arms.

Repeat *up to 10 times.*

---

* Watchpoints

– It is important to initiate the movement by lengthening and lifting your head first, and then your neck. When your head and neck are in line with your spine, you can then start to sequentially extend the upper spine.

– It is length not height that counts here, think long and strong to avoid compressing the spine.

Star

The Star teaches you how to move your limbs independent to a stable and extended upper spine. It also promotes strength and stamina in your upper back and shoulders essential for supporting the weight of heavy breasts and for carrying the baby! *Suitable for...* Preparing for Pregnancy, Pregnancy (up to 20 weeks), Postnatal. **Equipment** Folded towel (for forehead), small flat cushion (optional).

Starting position...

Lie on your front in a straight line. Rest your forehead on a folded towel. Legs are straight, slightly wider than hip-width and turned out from the hips. Reach both arms above your head, slightly wider than shoulder-width and resting on the mat, palms facing down. You may place a flat cushion underneath your abdomen to support your lower back.
Zip up to maintain a constant and appropriate connection to your centre throughout the exercise.

Action...

1 Breathe in, preparing your body to move, and, as you breathe out, lift your head and chest slightly off the mat to extend your upper spine.
2 Breathe in and lengthen your lifted spine.
3 Breathe out and, maintaining the position and stability of the spine, raise one arm and the opposite leg slightly off the mat.
4 Breathe in as you lower your arm and leg back down to the mat, again maintaining the lift and length of the upper body.
Repeat *actions 3 and 4 up to 10 times, lifting alternate arms and legs. Then lengthen and lower back down onto your mat.*

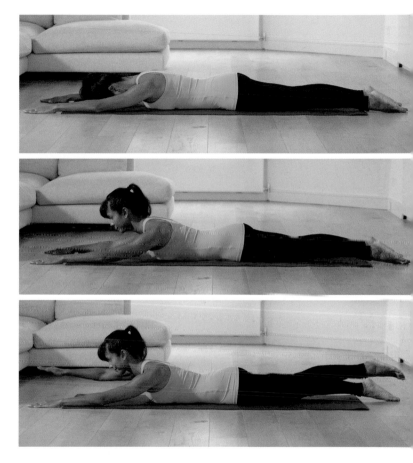

✳ Watchpoints

- Keep your core connected to support your lower back.
- Raise your arm and leg only as high as you can maintain a stable and still pelvis and spine.
- Keep your chest lifted away from the mat and the chest open. Your lower ribs should remain in contact with the mat and should also remain square; avoid any rocking in this area.
- Lengthen the arm forwards as it rises up, but avoid your shoulder over-elevating and creating tension.
- Fully lengthen your arms and legs but avoid locking your elbows and knees.

Table Top Stage 1

A great exercise for challenging the stability of the entire spine and shoulder girdle in a Four-point Kneeling position, while trying to find independent, free and flowing movement of opposing arms and legs. We have given you two stages to help you develop the relevant skills. *Suitable for...* All stages. Postnatal, wait for 6 weeks.

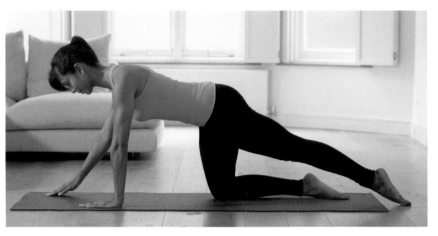

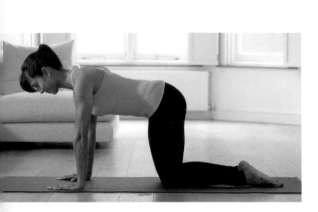

Starting position...
Four-point Kneeling.
Zip up to maintain a constant and appropriate connection to your centre throughout the exercise.

Action...
1 Breathe in to prepare your body to move and lengthen your spine.

2 Breathe out and maintaining a still and stable pelvis and spine, slide one leg behind you, directly in line with your hip. Simultaneously slide the opposite arm along the floor. Your softly pointed foot and your hand remain in contact with the mat.

3 Breathe in as you hold this lengthened position, ensuring that your spine does not dip in the middle.

4 Breathe out as you draw arm and leg back to the Starting position.

Repeat *up to 5 times on each side, then return to the Rest Position.*

Later pregnancy option
You may wish to place a large pillow, or bolster, between your knees, in readiness for when you come back into the Rest Position.

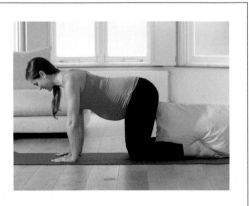

Table Top Stage 2

Suitable for... Preparing for Pregnancy only.

Follow the direction opposite up to Action point 3 then:

1 Breathe in as you lengthen and lift your leg to hip height. Simultaneously raise the opposite arm forwards, ideally to shoulder height.

2 Breathe out and lower your lengthened leg to the mat, and simultaneously return your arm underneath your shoulder.

3 Breathe in and once again maintaining neutral pelvis and spine slide your leg back in to the Starting position.

Repeat *up to 5 times on each side, alternating opposite arm and leg. Then return to the Rest Position.*

✳ Watchpoints

– Keep a good core connection to avoid your pelvis and spine dipping down towards the mat.

– Focus on the stability and stillness of your pelvis and ribcage as your leg moves freely and independently in the hip socket.

– Maintain a firm connection of the shoulder-blades to the back of your ribcage.

– Keep lengthening equally through both sides of the waist.

– Correctly co-ordinate the timing of your arm with your leg movement.

– Raise the arm to shoulder height, your leg to hip height, but only lift this high if you can maintain stillness in your pelvis and spine.

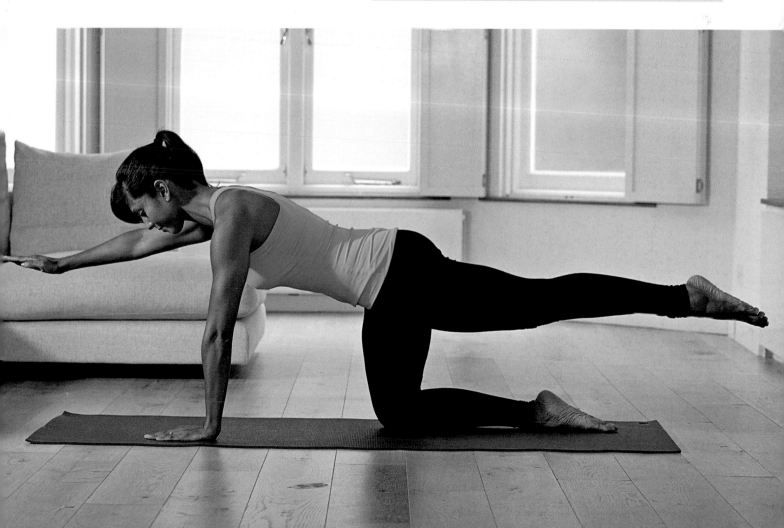

Rest Position

This is the perfect position to follow any back extension exercises such as Dart (page 94) or to follow a Four-point Kneeling exercise. The Rest Position gently stretches out your back while encouraging lateral breathing and release of the core, thus providing an opportunity to re-focus concentration in preparation for the next exercise. *Suitable for...* All stages.

Starting position...
Four-point Kneeling.

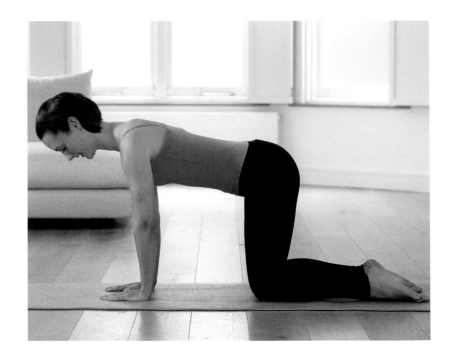

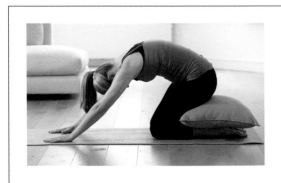

Early or later pregnancy option

Place a pillow under the thighs or between the knees and thighs, this avoids compressing the knee joints.

Alternatively a bolster works well between the knees, have another large pillow, or even a large ball to lean on (allowing bump room).

Note the different way to come out this position for Later Pregnancy: move back slowly into a Four-point Kneeling position before getting up, rather than sitting back on to your heels, restacking the spine.

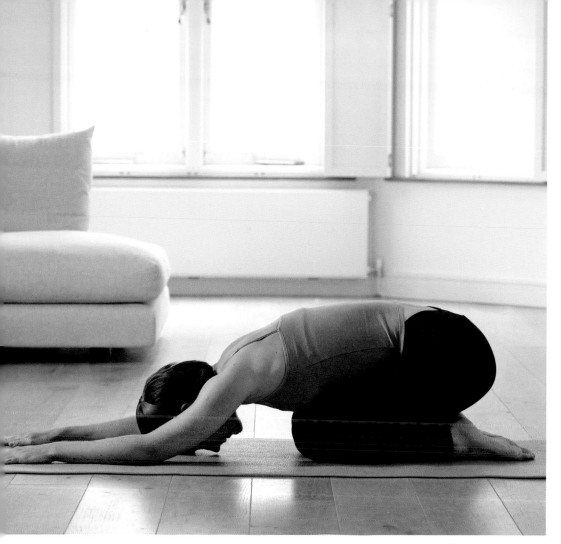

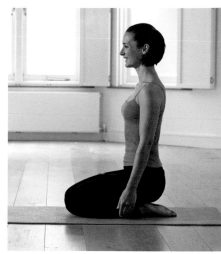

To finish...

Either: breathe out, zip up and begin by rolling your pelvis underneath you and then sequentially roll and restack your spine to an upright position, sitting back onto the heels. Or: for Later Pregnancy, breathe out, zip up and move forward back into Four-point Kneeling.

Action...

1 Breathe in, prepare your body, lengthen your spine and bring your feet slightly closer together.

2 Breathe out as you begin to fold at the hips and direct your buttocks backwards and down. Maintain the position of your hands on the mat and lengthen your arms. Ideally rest your sitting bones onto the heels or cushion, your chest onto the thighs and your forehead onto the mat (or pillow).

3 Breathe in and direct the breath into the back and the sides of your ribs and feel the ribcage progressively expand. You can allow your core muscles to relax.

4 Breathe out, fully emptying your lungs and focus on closing the ribs down and together.

Repeat *up to 10 times.*

✱ Watchpoints

– Avoid opening your knees too wide, the thighs should be slightly apart (which will allow bump room).
– Your head should feel supported (use a pillow if necessary) so that the neck can lengthen and relax.

Side Reach

A fabulous exercise which both stretches and strengthens your waist muscles. On a more technical note it encourages sequential lateral flexion of the spine. You have a choice of starting positions: Standing; Seated on a chair, mat or by a wall; Wall Slide Position; High Kneeling. The standing version is illustrated below, but choose whichever is most comfortable or you may vary the position for variety itself. *Suitable for...* All stages. Later Pregnancy choose whichever Starting position feels more comfortable. Take care not to overstretch especially if you know that you have a very large diastasis recti (abdominal divide).

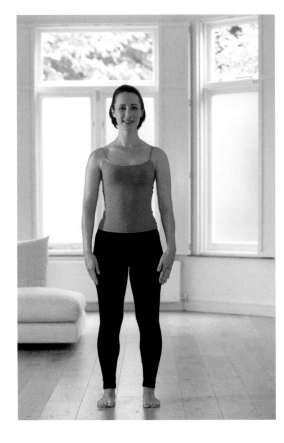

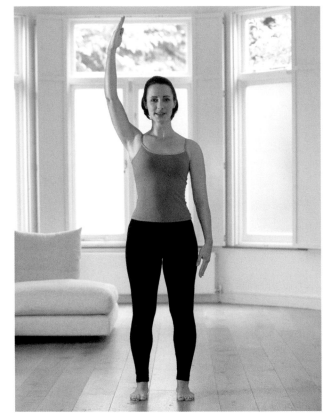

Starting position (standing)...

Stand tall on the floor, feet a little wider than hip-width apart to give you a wider base of support. Allow your arms to lengthen down by your sides.

Zip up to maintain a constant and appropriate connection to your centre throughout the exercise.

Action...

1 Breathe in as you raise your right arm out to the side and overhead.

2 Breathe out as you reach up and over, leading with your head, sequentially bending your spine to the left. If sitting on a mat, your left arm will reactively slide further along the mat and then bend, so that your forearm can support your position. If standing, your left arm will remain lengthened and slide down the outside of your left leg.

3 Breathe in. Maintain the length and position of your spine and focus on breathing into your open side.

4 Breathe out as you lengthen the spine back to upright. Lower your right arm down by your side.

Repeat *up to 5 times to each side.*

❋ Watchpoints

– As you reach over, initiate the movement with an incline of your head and continue moving through your neck and then your ribcage. Reverse the sequence as you return to the upright position, always maintaining length in your spine and focusing on the connection to your centre.

– As you reach, maintain the relationship between the arm and your head, do not allow the shoulder to hike up.

– Lengthen up through both sides of your waist as you stretch.

– Moved in one plane only – sideways, do not curve forward or arch back.

– Keep your head and neck in line with the rest of your spine, your gaze remains forward.

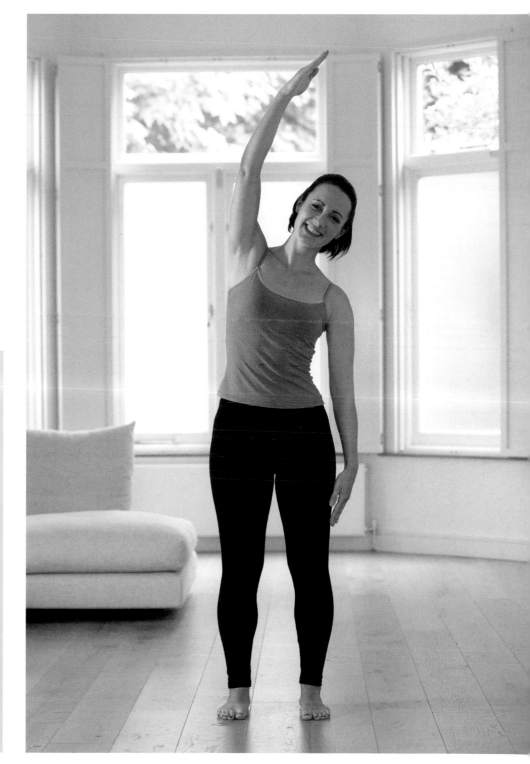

Roll Downs

A favourite due to its feel-good factor, this exercise is a winner as it helps to mobilise the spine and hips, strengthening the muscles of your back, buttocks and legs as they allow you to bend forwards with control. *Suitable for...* Preparing for Pregnancy, Early Pregnancy (but take care that you do not feel dizzy due to lowered blood pressure, you may prefer to use the wall as described below). Postnatal.

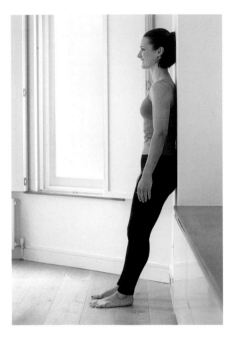

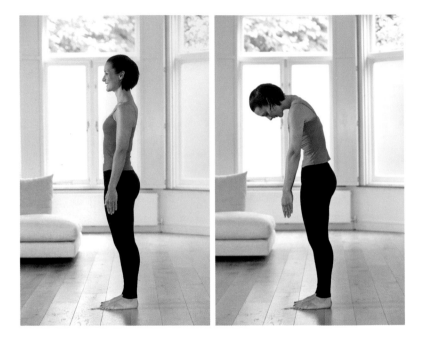

Practice Roll Downs...

You may practise Roll Downs by using a wall for guidance. Stand tall with your back against a wall. Place your feet in parallel and hip-width apart, approximately 30–60cm from the wall and bend your knees ever so slightly. In this position your pelvis is in neutral and should feel supported by the wall. Your spine is also in neutral so you will feel its natural curves. The back of the head may or may not be in contact depending on your individual posture. Allow your arms to lengthen down by the sides of your body. Then follow the Action points below.

Starting position...

Stand tall on the floor, your feet in parallel and hip-width apart, and bend your knees ever so slightly. **Zip up to maintain a constant and appropriate connection to your centre throughout the exercise.**

Action...

1 Breathe in as you lengthen the back of your neck and nod your head forwards.

2 Breathe out as you continue to roll your spine forwards, softening your breastbone and wheeling your spine as far as you can, then bend from hips to go as far as comfortable.

3 Breathe in as you begin to roll your pelvis underneath you.

4 Breathe out as you continue to roll your spine back up, restacking each vertebra until you stand up tall.

Repeat *up to 5 times.*

✳ Watchpoints

– Ensure that you roll smoothly and sequentially through each segment of your spine.

– As you roll down, begin the movement with a nod of your head and as you roll up, begin the movement from your pelvis rolling underneath.

– Roll directly through your centreline avoiding any deviations to either side.

– Keep your weight balanced evenly on both feet. Also, do not allow your feet to roll either in or out.

– Create space between each vertebra, imagine you are stretching up and over a large beach ball.

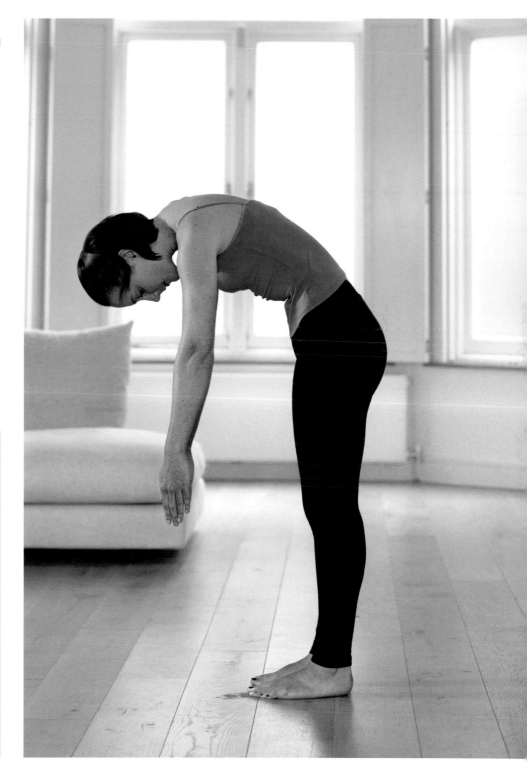

Pelvic Floor Control

We've done the groundwork already in 'The Bottom Line' on page 24 where we explained the importance of pelvic floor control. In the chapter on Centring (pages 58) we introduced you to The Wind Zip and showed you how it can be used to help with stability.

Here we are going to focus completely and only on the pelvic floor, although the action of The Wind Zip is still appropriate as you will see. This does not mean that your abdominal muscles do not join in, they cannot help it, but your focus this time is on the pelvic floor itself.

* Watchpoints

– Ensure that you do not pull up or in too hard. It is very important that you do not force this pelvic floor action or grip.

– Make sure that you keep your buttock muscles relaxed. Your pelvis remains still throughout, the action of the elevator is purely internal.

– Keep your chest and the front of your shoulders open and avoid any tension in your neck area.

– Continue to breathe fully throughout; it is very important not to hold your breath.

– If you lose any of the connections, relax and start again from the beginning.

– On the way down with the lift, ensure that your mouth and jaw are relaxed.

First some pelvic floor facts:

* Pelvic floor exercises are best done in frequent batches of about six contractions at a time.

* Try to focus on drawing up every muscle fibre – it is the quality of the contraction that counts.

* Never hold your breath while contracting the pelvic floor.

* Do not be tempted to practise your pelvic floor exercises while on the toilet. The toilet seat puts your pelvis at the wrong angle. You may practise them, however, sitting with the lid down!

* Try to do your pelvic floor exercises regularly throughout the day – while waiting at traffic lights, while queuing etc.

* If you have trouble locating your pelvic floor you can try sucking your thumb!

* Different cues and different positions suit different mothers.

* Experiment with the following exercises in a variety of positions: see what works for you.

* Remember to do some pelvic floor release work too.

Starting position...

Sit tall on a chair. Place your feet on the floor, hip-width apart or connecting your inner thighs together. Make sure that your weight is even on both sitting bones and that your spine is lengthened in neutral.

Imagine that your pelvic floor is a lift in a building. This exercise requires you to take the 'lift' up to different floors of the building; three floors to be precise. Don't climb up too far too quickly or you will run out of floors! The grand finale is descending down into the basement. Try to completely release your pelvic floor. Experiment and see if it helps you to do this finale decent on an in-breath.

The Pelvic Elevator

This commonly used exercise helps you to identify degrees of pelvic floor contraction and also introduces release in stages (on the way down). *Suitable for...* All stages.

Action...

1 Breathe wide in and lengthen your spine.

2 Breathe out and gently Wind Zip back to front visualising gently sliding the doors of the lift shut.

3 Breathe in and hold the doors closed.

4 Breathe out and take the lift to the first floor of the building.

5 Breathe in and focus on keeping the lift on the first floor with the doors shut. This will help you to gently maintain the connection of your pelvic floor muscles.

6 Breathe out as you slowly take the lift up, a little higher to the second floor. Engage your pelvic floor muscles slightly more.

7 Breathe in and hold the lift on the second floor.

8 Breathe out as you take the lift to the third floor. Gently engage your pelvic floor muscles even more but avoid over-gripping.

9 Breathe in as you hold the lift on the third floor.

10 Breathe out as you slowly lower the lift back down a floor.

11 Repeat this descent floor by floor until your reach the ground floor.

12 Then breathe in and as you breathe out allow the lift to descend to the basement floor, allow the doors to slide open.

13 Breathe in and as you breathe out just gently slide the doors closed again. Ready to start again…

Repeat *up to 3 times.*

Pillow Squeeze

This is a very useful exercise for isolating the pelvic floor. Sometimes, even with practice, we can grip the inner thigh muscles instead of the pelvic floor. *Suitable for...* All stages.

* Watchpoints

– It is very important that you allow your mouth to remain soft and released as you do these exercises.

– If you like, you may softly blow through your mouth as you release the pelvic floor.

– It helps to blow against your hand.

– Keep an eye out too for unwanted tension in the calves!

Later pregnancy option

You may use Seated on a Chair as your start position, again with a small pillow between your thighs.

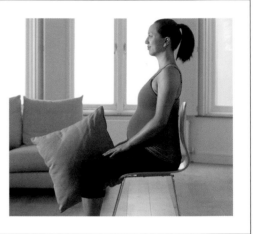

Starting position...
The Relaxation Position. Place a small pillow between your thighs.

Action...

1 Breathe in to prepare.

2 Breathe out as you Wind Zip.

3 Breathe in and hold the zip.

4 Breathe out and, still Wind Zipping, add a gently squeeze to the pillow.

5 Breathe in and release your Wind Zip, keep the pillow squeeze.

6 Breathe out and release your pillow squeeze.

Repeat *up to 4 times.* **Then reverse it...**

1 Breathe in to prepare.

2 Breathe out as you squeeze the pillow gently.

3 Breathe in and hold the squeeze.

4 Breathe out and add a Wind Zip.

5 Breathe in and release your pillow squeeze.

6 Breathe out and release your Wind Zip.

Repeat *up to 4 times.*

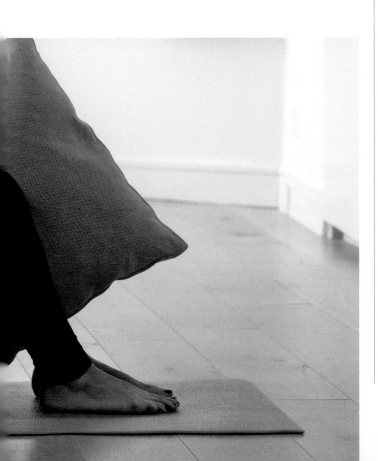

The Emergency Stop

Stress incontinence is surprisingly common during and following pregnancy. The following exercise will help you to cope with emergencies such as coughing or sneezing, when you may not have the time to go up all the floors of the lift! *Suitable for...* All stages.

Starting position...

You may pick your favourite! But it's probably easiest seated.

Action...

1 Breathe normally, simply lift the whole of the pelvic floor, tightening it all quickly as if in an emergency.

2 Hold for about five seconds, keep breathing, breathing… then release.

Practise *6 times.*

> **✱ Watchpoints**
> – Try to only engage your pelvic floor and not your jaw, neck, shoulders, buttocks and thighs!

Breathing and the Pelvic Floor

In this exercise we will be using deep abdominal breathing to help calm your mind and also to help you relax all your muscles, especially those around the abdomen and pelvic floor. This is an important counterbalance to all the zipping up we will be doing! If you can make some sounds with your out-breath it will help to prepare you for releasing sounds on the out-breath during labour where it may help you manage your contractions. *Suitable for...* All stages.

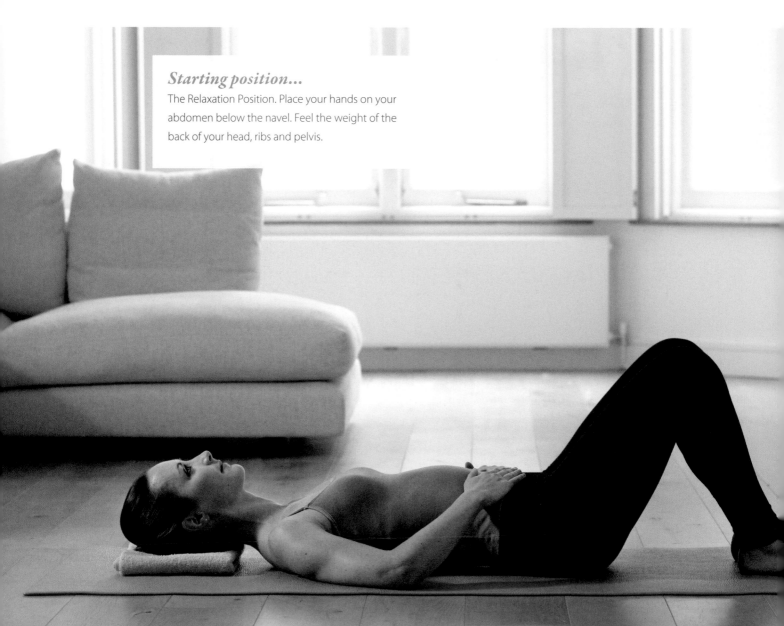

Starting position...
The Relaxation Position. Place your hands on your abdomen below the navel. Feel the weight of the back of your head, ribs and pelvis.

Action...

1 Bring your focus onto your breathing, become aware of the rhythm of its ebb and flow.

2 Breathe in through your nose and out through your mouth, letting your jaw and throat soften.

3 After each out-breath, take a moment's pause before you breathe in again.

4 Allow each out-breath to lengthen until your out-breath is about twice as long as your in-breath.

5 Now move your awareness down to your abdomen.

6 Notice what happens as you breathe in. Feel how your abdomen expands.

7 Feel how the abdomen draws away from your hands as you breathe out. Continue observing this gentle movement in the abdomen.

8 Breathe deep down into the abdomen and pelvis.

9 Breathe out from the base of your pelvis. Allow the rest of your body to remain soft and open.

10 When you feel ready, try making some sounds as you breathe out, a sigh perhaps, an 'ahh' sound, or whatever comes naturally.

Early or later pregnancy option

Seated, with or without your back to the wall, using whatever pillows you need to make yourself feel comfortable. Close your eyes, lengthen the back of your neck and allow your head to nod gently forwards. Allow your collar-bones and shoulders to widen. If seated, feel your sitting bones grounded, your back supported. Gently cup your bump. NB you can also use this starting position if you are not pregnant, if you prefer.

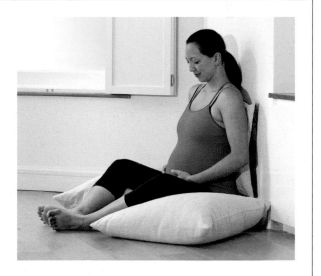

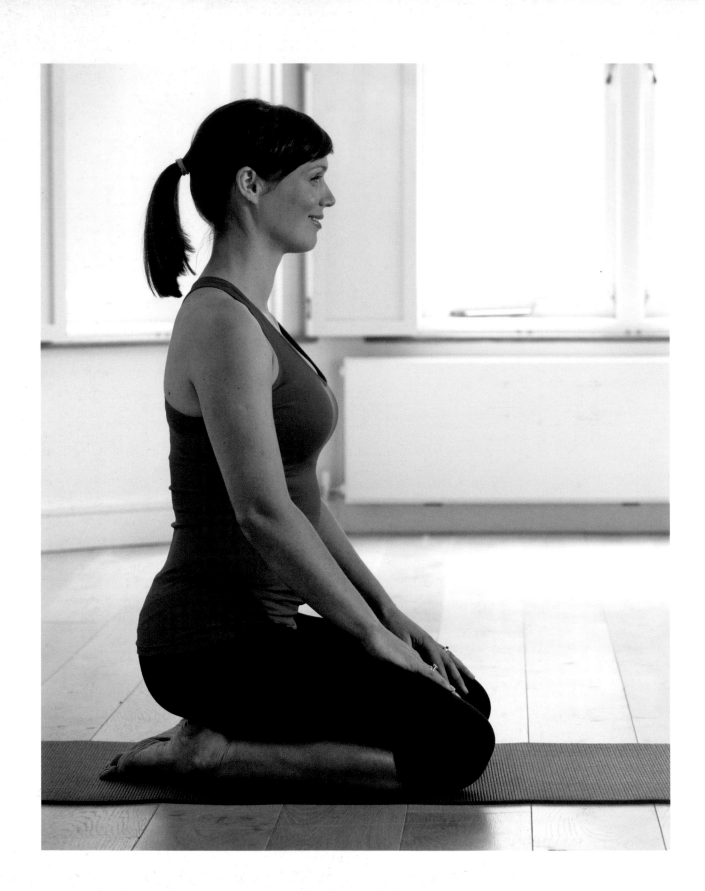

The Early Pregnancy Programme

3

The Early Pregnancy Programme

Remember that only mothers who have been regularly practising Pilates for at least four months should follow this programme.

It is essential that you obtain your practitioner's permission to continue to exercise at regular intervals throughout your pregnancy.

Your changing body (0–16 weeks)

Over the next few weeks, your body's priority is to build your baby's life support system. This is going to require lots of energy so it's no wonder you may be feeling tired and sleepy. Your heart rate is increased, your blood sugar has dropped, your metabolic rate is burning lots of energy. You are not ill, this is a normal state for women, but you do need to take things easy.

There is a lot of pressure on women these days to be superwoman, to continue to work and be a domestic goddess. You may feel fantastic and perfectly able to carry on as before. But listen to what your body is telling you: if you need rest, you need rest. The high levels of progesterone in your body can have a sedative effect, making you feel more sleepy. We have already seen (page 15) how the increase in your blood volume may lead to blood dilution anaemia which may make you feel extra tired. You need once again to balance work, play, activity and rest.

This does not mean that you have to stop exercising. It would be a shame to waste these early weeks as they provide the perfect opportunity for you to maintain your well-earned movement skills and all the health benefits of Pilates. But it does mean that you should consider carefully when and how you exercise. Your exercise priorities need to change to take into account what is happening inside.

Most women feel their first pregnancy symptoms around 6 weeks. About half of women experience nausea during their pregnancy, it is most common between 6 and 16 weeks but can come back later in pregnancy. Generally called morning sickness, it can, for some unlucky women, last all day! Do not worry, pregnancy nausea is not thought to affect the development of your baby. But whenever you feel able to eat, try to eat as healthily as possible and be sure to include plenty of micronutrient-rich food (e.g. fresh vegetables, especially green ones) to provide all the vitamins and minerals needed to help build your baby's organs. Check too that you are drinking enough fluids and keep an eye on your weight; if it starts to drop because you cannot eat properly, do tell your doctor (see opposite for advice on weight gain).

Some pregnant women have a lot of saliva and some report a metallic taste in the mouth. You may find your appetite affected by cravings for some foods and aversion to others. Within reason, and common sense, trust your body's instincts. My mother had wanted to eat coal with me! Soap and tomatoes with my brother!

Your breasts might feel different already. If you have been pregnant before you will recognise the change in that your breasts are more sensitive, fuller and tingly. Breasts can leak colostrum from as early as 16 weeks. Your sense of smell is heightened. You will probably need to pass urine a lot, due to the increased metabolic rate, but not all women find this, some find they need to go less. Be sure you are drinking enough fluids to keep you hydrated, but don't overdo it. Remember, there is water in food, especially fruits and vegetables. There is varying advice on how much water, 6–8 glasses a day is often advised, but much depends on what you are eating, the weather and what you are doing and your own metabolism. Your urine should be pale in colour.

Unfortunately your hormones may make you prone to urinary tract infections (cystitis). Your pelvic organs are changing position, and the lengthening of the urethra and pushing up of the bladder by the growing uterus sometimes prevent the bladder from emptying properly, so causing urine to become stagnant. Drinking enough water can help here too, as can remembering to urinate after intercourse. Avoid wearing tight jeans and restrictive exercise clothes as they can aggravate the condition. If you feel any discomfort when passing water, do tell your doctor as, left untreated, cystitis can go on to become a kidney infection which is more serious. Keeping hydrated and eating well will also help you to avoid the other common condition of pregnancy, constipation, and its constant companions, bloating, indigestion and wind.

You may experience dramatic mood swings, up one minute, down the next, you may be irritable and over-sensitive, feelings often associated with premenstrual tension. You may find you are getting headaches and feeling occasionally dizzy. That is fine, but severe headaches or dizziness need immediate medical attention (see page 29).

Our focus in this Early Pregnancy Programme is to reinforce and maintain all the mind/body awareness, relaxation and movement skills you have learnt in the Preparing for Pregnancy Programme. Stability work for all the joints is high on our list of priorities due to the ligamentous laxity. Exercises for your posture, breathing and pelvic floor control are also included. We want to keep you supple but with an inner strength and to maintain the equilibrium you hopefully achieved by following the Preparing for Pregnancy Programme or in your Pilates classes.

Between 14 and 16 weeks, most women first feel the baby move inside – this is called the quickening and is a truly memorable moment. From now on you will start to feel the baby flexing its own muscles as he or she experiments with their own fitness techniques such as somersaulting, football, cycling. The strangest feeling

of all is if your baby gets the hiccups! Later on in your pregnancy, the baby will have grown so much that there is less room for manoeuvre.

Around 16 weeks, your baby's life support, the placenta, will be complete, and your body will settle down. Hopefully the nausea will cease (not always) and you will be more adjusted to all the hormonal changes. Time then to move on to The Later Pregnancy Programme.

Weight gain during pregnancy

A lot of mothers become concerned with their weight during pregnancy. Just how much weight should you gain? Should you be eating for two?

While it is important to keep an eye on your weight gain, you must not become overly anxious about it. Your midwife will check your weight when you visit the antenatal clinic and let you know if you are off course. Try not to compare yourself with other mothers to be. The amount of weight gained during pregnancy varies enormously from woman to woman and pregnancy to pregnancy. Remember too that only some of your weight gain is due to increased body fat. The rest is your unborn baby, the placenta, the amniotic fluid and the increase in maternal blood and fluid volume.

Your practitioner will probably give you an indication as to how much weight you should gain during your pregnancy. This is going to vary according to:
– Your height
– Your pre-pregnancy weight and BMI (see page 76)
– How many babies you are having.

During the first trimester most women gain about 0.9–1.8kg. The rate at which you gain weight usually increases during your second trimester and then it may slow down again in the third. As the due date gets nearer, most women stop gaining weight.

The pattern of your weight gain or weight loss is a good indicator as to how your pregnancy is progressing. Evidence suggests that there is an increased risk of maternal health problems during pregnancy if you are over- or underweight. There is also evidence to suggest that low birth-weight babies are more prone to health problems later in life, especially those whose mothers followed a diet low in nutrients in the early months of pregnancy when the baby's organs were being formed.

There is no need for you to eat for two but you will need some extra calories, about 300 extra calories per day for the second and third trimesters. The final birth weight of your baby will be related to a number of factors including genetics, your metabolic rate and the efficiency of the placenta (the exception being diabetic mothers). There are different views as to the precise impact your diet has on your baby's birth weight and later health but it makes good sense to try to eat a varied and healthy balanced diet from the moment you decide to start a family right through your postnatal months and beyond.

By the end of your pregnancy, if you are of average weight and build, the normal recommendation is that you gain between 11.25–16kg.

If you find that you are suddenly losing weight, then seek medical advice.

The gentle exercise programme in this book will certainly help you to manage your weight, keeping you active but note that exercise should not be used to lose weight during pregnancy.

Exercise guidelines for the first 16 weeks

Before you exercise, take a moment to stop and listen to your body. Use your intuition. Ask yourself, is this the right time for me to exercise? If it feels right do only what you feel comfortable doing. Trust your instincts.

* Try to include some relaxation exercises as often as you can.

* Take your time getting down onto the mat and up again. Always roll over onto your side and wait a moment before getting up.

* Standing exercises are fine but avoid standing still for too long.

* You may find that exercises such as Roll Downs make you dizzy, if so, avoid!

* Pay close attention to your alignment both when you are getting into your Starting positions and while you are doing the exercises.

* Quality of movement, not quantity counts.

* Take care not to overstretch or overwork your abdominal muscles.

* Avoid exercises which involve taking your weight onto one leg.

* Avoid overstretching and holding stretches for long periods of time.

* If you get confused with the breathing pattern, or if you run out of breath, just keep breathing, and use your own natural rhythm.

* Do your pelvic floor exercises regularly, daily if possible. Be sure to include some release work.

* Include plenty of pelvic stability exercises, revisit The Fundamentals, such as Leg Slides and Single Knee Folds. But avoid the more challenging exercises, such as Double Knee Folds.

* Take your Pilates class with you wherever you go. Remember good posture as you go about your daily activities. See page 142.

Early Pregnancy Workouts

As well as the exercises listed in this chapter, you will also be able to add to your workouts the following exercises from the rest of the book:

– All the exercises from Preparing for Pregnancy except the Single Leg Stretch.

– All the exercises for Later Pregnancy and Preparing for the Birth.

From the Postnatal Exercise Programme:

– Cobra Prep (page 207)

– Crawling Lizard (page 208)

– Spine Curls with Support (page 199)

– Ribcage Closure and Leg Slide (page 202)

If you design your own workouts, try to include some spinal flexion, rotation, side flexion and extension. Balance upper and lower body work too. Here are two sample workouts for you to try.

Workout One

Relaxation Position . . . . *(page 40)*
Knee Circles . . . . *(page 120)*
Nose Spirals . . . . *(page 117)*
Starfish . . . . *(page 70)*
Spine Curls with Ribcage Closure . . . . *(page 82)*
Curl Ups with Knee Extension . . . . *(page 84)*
Hip Rolls . . . . *(page 93)*
Oyster . . . . *(page 161)*
Side-lying Circles . . . . *(page 166)*
Arm Openings . . . . *(page 160)*
Diamond Press . . . . *(page 122)*
Dart . . . . *(page 94)*
Oblique Cat into Rest Position . . . . *(page 125)*

Pelvic Floor Control (seated on mat) . . . . *(page 104)*
Side Reach (standing) . . . . *(page 100)*
Waist Twist (standing) . . . . *(page 126)*
Tennis Ball Rising . . . . *(page 127)*
Roll Downs (on the wall) – watch for dizziness . . *(page 102)*

Workout Two

Wall Slides A or B . . . . *(pages 36–39)*
Floating Arms . . . . *(page 66)*
Dumb Waiter Variation . . . . *(page 157)*
Waist Twist (standing) . . . . *(page 126)*
Shoulder Drops Variation . . . . *(page 81)*
Pillow Squeeze . . . . *(page 106)*
Pelvic Stability Variation . . . . *(page 118)*
Spine Curls . . . . *(page 58)*
Curl Ups with Knee Openings . . . . *(page 84)*
Star Variation . . . . *(page 123)*
Cobra Prep . . . . *(page 207)*
Cat . . . . *(page 124)*
Rest Position . . . . *(page 98)*
Arm Openings . . . . *(page 160)*
Pelvic Floor Control (seated on chair) . . . . *(page 104)*
Foot exercises . . . . *(pages 128–131)*
Side Reach . . . . *(page 100)*
Ribcage Closure (in Wall Slide) . . . . *(page 69)*
Pilates Squat . . . . *(page 153)*

Knee Rolls

In this exercise you will be rolling the thigh bones on the pelvis to help mobilise the hip. Yet you must still maintain a stable relationship between the hip, knee and ankle joints. It also challenges the stability of your spine as the legs move independently from the hips.
Suitable for... Preparing for Pregnancy, Early Pregnancy, Postnatal.

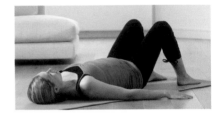

Starting position...

The Relaxation Position. Position your legs slightly wider than hip-width apart. Place your hands onto your pelvis to check for unwanted movement if you wish or you can reach your arms out on the mat slightly lower than shoulder height with your palms facing down.
Zip up to maintain a constant and appropriate connection to your centre throughout the exercise.

Action...

1 Breathe in to prepare your body to move.

2 Breathe out as you roll your right leg in from the hip joint and simultaneously roll the left leg out, also from the hip joint. Both knees will therefore roll to the left; allow your feet to roll with the movement. Try to keep your pelvis relatively still.

3 Breathe in and return both legs back to the centre at the same time.

Repeat *to the other side and then repeat the whole sequence up to 5 times.*

Nose Spirals

Once you've tried this exercise you will appreciate why it is so popular. It's perfect for when you are feeling stressed as it helps release tension. *Suitable for...* Preparing for Pregnancy, Early Pregnancy, Postnatal. Later Pregnancy: you can use any seated position. Just take care that your head does not tip back. Your head is moving on top of your spine, your neck actually stays almost still.

Starting position...
The Relaxation Position.
You may give your core muscles a break for this exercise.

Action...
Breathe naturally throughout. Keeping your neck lengthened and released, begin to roll your head in a small spiralling motion. Allow each circle to be slightly larger than the last. After about 10 circles, start to spiral the other way in ever-decreasing circles.

Later pregnancy option
Later Pregnancy mothers try seated on a chair (you will need to be near the front of the chair)

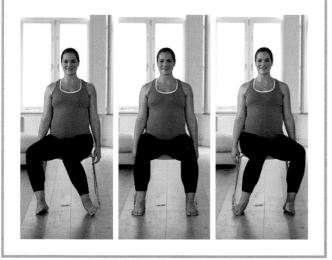

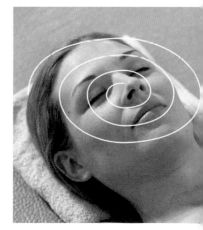

Pelvic Stability Variation

Starting position...

The Relaxation Position. Hold the band or scarf above your shoulders, wrists and fingers long.

Zip up to maintain a constant and appropriate connection to your centre throughout the exercise.

Now, more than ever, you need to reinforce your natural corset by working on your pelvic stability. This is a variation along that theme, combining several exercises, Shoulder Drops, Ribcage Closure, and Knee Folds with an added Leg Extension for good measure. *Suitable for...* Preparing for Pregnancy, Early Pregnancy and Postnatal only. **Equipment** A stretch band or scarf.

Preparation Action...

1 Breathe in and reach both arms up to the ceiling, allowing your shoulder-blades to lift from the mat as for Shoulder Drops.

2 Breathe out and slowly replace both shoulder-blades on the mat, widening your collar-bones and releasing your neck.

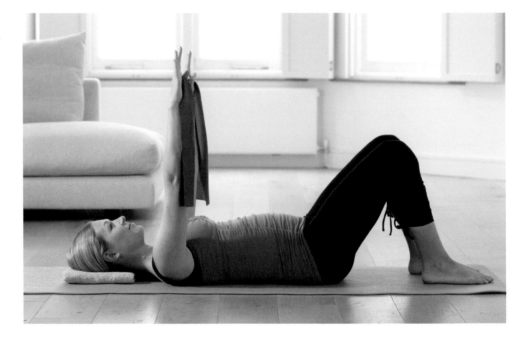

✳ Watchpoints

– Use your core to help prevent the ribs flaring or the lower back arching.

– Visualise your strong centre, just below the navel so that you can focus on your limbs lengthening away from this point.

– Try to keep the movements controlled and flowing. Co-ordinate your movements to help improve your spatial awareness.

– Use your breath to help the flow.

– Take care not to lower the leg too far as the weight of the leg may pull your lower back into an over-arched position.

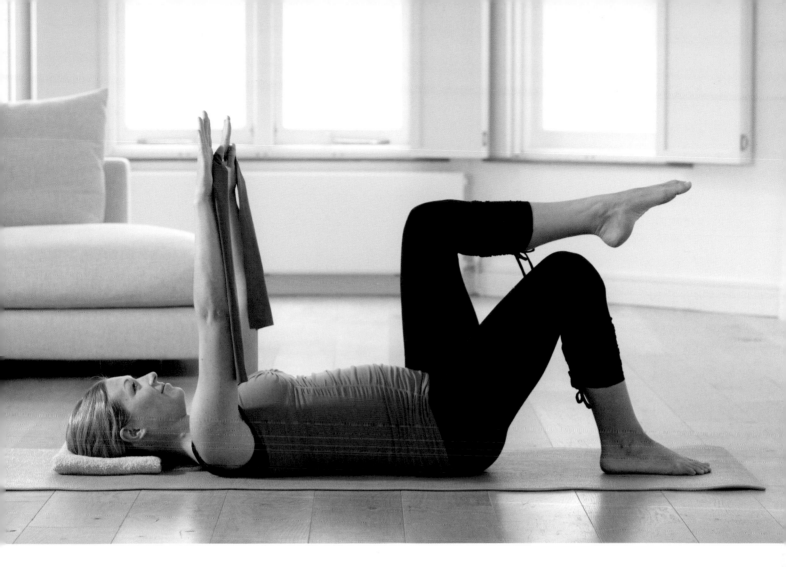

Main Action...

1 Breathe in and fold your left leg in towards you without disturbing your pelvis.

2 Breathe out and slowly straighten your leg at about a 45 degree angle, while simultaneously taking both arms behind you in a Ribcage Closure movement.

3 Breathe in and fold your leg back in towards you, bringing your arms back in line with your shoulders.

4 Breathe out and replace the foot on the mat.

Repeat *up 5 times with each leg, before lowering the arms back down by your sides.*

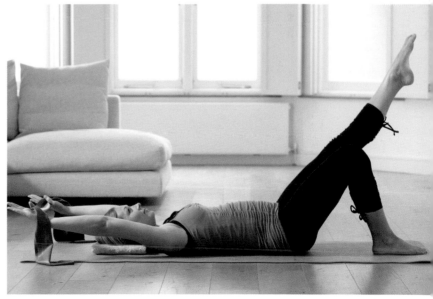

Knee Circles

Like Knee Rolls, this exercise helps you to learn how to move your thigh bone independently of your pelvis and spine. The ability to do so will help release tension around the hip joint while also improving spinal stability. *Suitable for...* Preparing for Pregnancy, Early Pregnancy and Postnatal.

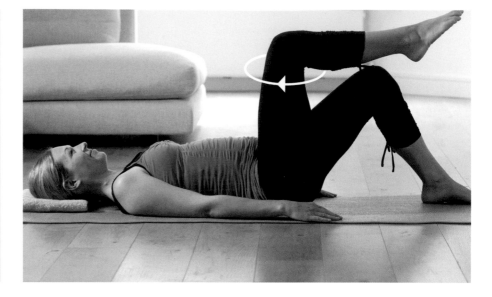

✳ Watchpoints

– Keep your pelvis and spine stable and still throughout; focus on the independent movement of the thigh bone in the hip socket.

– The supporting leg should be still but free from tension.

– Keep your chest and the front of your shoulders open and neck released.

– Begin with small circles, about the size of a grapefruit, and work up to larger circles, watermelons, as you learn to gain more control.

Starting position...

The Relaxation Position. Fold one leg in towards your body with stability.

Zip up to maintain a constant and appropriate connection to your centre throughout the exercise.

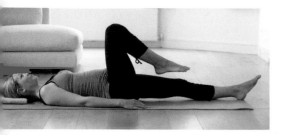

Action...

1 Breathing naturally and at your own pace, begin to circle your leg towards the midline of the body and then continue to circle the leg down, around and back up to the Starting position. Draw your leg in as close to the body as is possible without disturbing the pelvis.

Repeat *up to 5 times and then reverse the direction.*

2 To finish, return your knee so that it is in line with the hip joint and then, maintaining a stable pelvis return your leg to the mat to finish in the Relaxation Position.

Repeat *with the other leg, up to 5 times in each direction.*

Variation

When you have mastered this version, try the slightly more challenging version where the non-circling leg is stretched out along the mat in line with the hip. Take care that your pelvis remains in neutral. The circling leg may relax from the knee down to allow you to focus on the movement happening at the hip itself.

Curl Ups with Leg Extension

We do not want to overstretch your hamstrings at the back of your thighs, but we want to keep them lengthened. The leg extension element of the exercise is a safe way to do this as you use the dynamic movement to gently stretch them out. *Suitable for...* Preparing for Pregnancy, Early Pregnancy and Postnatal (once the abdominal muscle divide has improved to 2cm or less and there is no bulging).

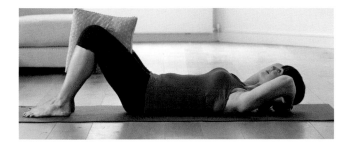

Starting position...

The Relaxation Position. Place a cushion between your knees, Lightly clasp both hands behind your head, keeping the elbows open and positioned just in front of your ears, within your peripheral vision.

Zip up to maintain a constant and appropriate connection to your centre throughout the exercise.

> ## ✳ **Watchpoints**
> – Keep your pelvis centred.
> – The pillow is there to guide you and keep a gentle connection between your legs. Do not squeeze it.
> – Focus on wheeling your spine off the mat vertebra by vertebra; remember that curling back down sequentially is just as important.
> – Allow your head to be supported in your hands, your neck free from tension.
> – Lengthen the leg away but at the same time keep it anchored in your hip.

Action...

1 Breathe in, preparing your body to move.

2 Breathe out as you nod your head and curl up from the mat, simultaneously straightening one leg from the knee, the cushion stays put.

3 Breathe into the back of the ribs to maintain the curled up position.

4 Breathe out as you slowly curl back down with control, while bending the knee and replacing your foot on the mat.

Repeat, *straightening alternate legs up to 5 times with each leg.*

Diamond Press

Probably one of our best exercises for correcting poor posture. It really helps to mobilise and strengthen muscles of the upper spine and gently lengthens you out. *Suitable for...* Preparing for Pregnancy, Pregnancy as long as you feel comfortable lying on your front (or 20 weeks, whichever is sooner), Postnatal. If you are going to finish by coming back into the Rest Position, have any pillows you may need nearby.

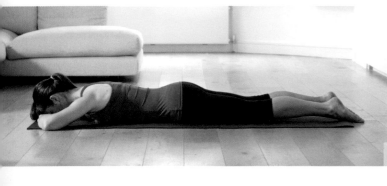

Starting position...

Lie on your front in a straight line. Create a diamond shape with the arms: place the fingertips together, palms down onto the mat and open your elbows. Rest your forehead on the backs of the hands. Your legs are hip-width apart and parallel. (You may place a pillow under your shins if it helps you feel more comfortable.)

Zip up to maintain a constant and appropriate connection to your centre throughout the exercise.

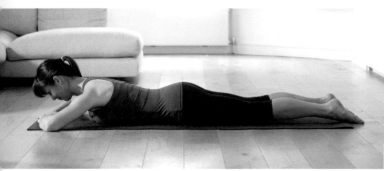

Action...

1   Breathe in to prepare.

2   Breathe out as you lift first your head, then your neck and then your chest off the mat. Feel your lower ribs remaining in contact with the mat, but open your chest and focus on directing it forwards.

3   Breathe in as you hold this position.

4   Breathe out as you return first your chest and head sequentially back down to the mat with control.

Repeat *up to 10 times, then, unless you are doing another Back Extension exercise, finish by coming up into Four-point Kneeling, then if you can, come back into Rest Position.*

✳ Watchpoints

–   Start the movement by lengthening, then lifting your head first, and then your neck follows. When your head and neck are in line with the rest of your spine you can begin to open and lift your chest.

–   Keep your lower ribs in contact with the mat as you lift up; this will ensure that you do not lift too far. It is length not height that we are aiming for.

–   Keep your core engaged to support your spine.

–   Avoid too much pressure down into the arms; they are there to lightly support you and not to press you up.

–   Keep your feet in contact with the mat throughout (unless you have used an extra pillow).

Star Variation

This exercise is a combination of Star and Diamond Press. It uses movement skills from both. As well as being great for your posture, it also works the buttocks (which can get somewhat flabby during pregnancy). *Suitable for...* Preparing for Pregnancy, Pregnancy up to 20 weeks only, Postnatal. If you are going to finish by coming back into the Rest Position, have any pillows you may need nearby.

Starting position...

Lie on your front, legs turned out from the hips just wider than hip-width apart. Fold your left arm so you can rest your forehead on it. Stretch the right arm out so it is just wider than shoulder-width. Maintain a distance between the ears and the shoulders. Keep a sense of openness in the upper body.

Zip up to maintain a constant and appropriate connection to your centre throughout the exercise.

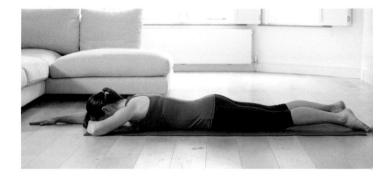

Action...

1   Breathe in to prepare and lengthen through the spine.

2   Breathe out as you lengthen and lift your head and chest slightly off the mat, lifting your left arm with you. Simultaneously lengthen and lift the right leg a few centimetres off the floor, only as high as you do not disturb the pelvis.

3   Breathe in and hold this lengthened position.

4   Breathe out and lengthen through the whole body as you lower your chest, head, arm and leg.

Repeat up to 5 times then change arms so that your right arm is supporting your head and repeat up to 5 more times, lifting the left leg. Then, unless you are doing another back extension exercise, finish by coming up into Four-point Kneeling, then if you can come back into Rest Position.

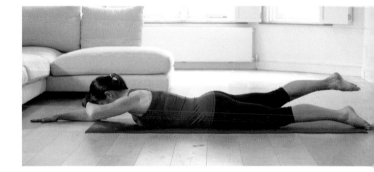

✳ Watchpoints

–   Your lower ribs stay in contact with the mat.

–   Avoid compressing your lower back by keeping your core muscles engaged.

–   Do not push yourself up with the resting arm, your mid-back muscles need to work.

–   Your head stays in contact with the back of your hand but should not feel heavy there.

–   Maintain distance between your ears and your shoulders, do not allow them to creep up.

–   Keep both hips on the mat, pelvis stable, the thigh bone really lengthening and reaching out of the hip joint.

–   The most common mistake is to lift the leg too high.

The Cat

This will be a favourite throughout your pregnancy. It takes pressure off your spine and gently mobilises it, helping to release tension. Remember the gentle upper back extension you learnt with Diamond Press – it's the same subtle movement here. The variation adds extra work for your oblique abdominals. *Suitable for...* All stages. Caution in the first few weeks postnatal.

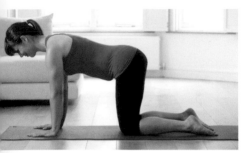

Starting position...

Four-point Kneeling.

Zip up to maintain a constant and appropriate connection to your centre throughout the exercise.

Action...

1 Breathe in to prepare your body, lengthen your spine.

2 Breathe out as you roll your pelvis underneath you as if directing your tailbone between your legs. As you do so, your lower back will gently round, continue this movement allowing your upper back to also round, followed by your neck, and finally nod your head slightly forwards. This position is an even and balanced 'C' shape of the spine.

3 Breathe in wide to the lower ribcage to help maintain this lengthened 'C 'shape.

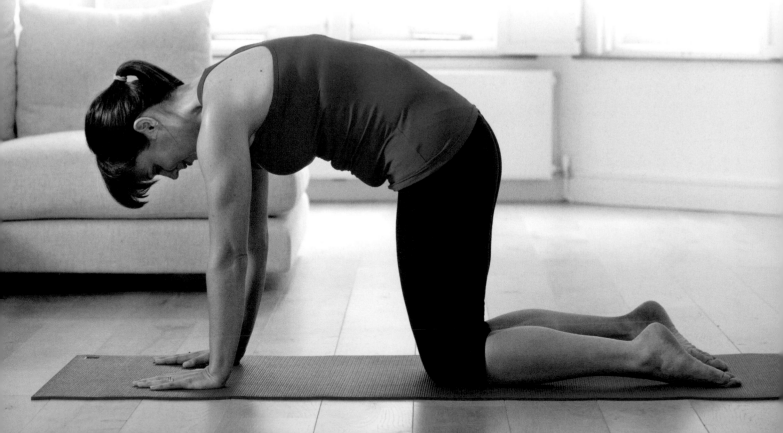

4 Breathe out as you simultaneously start to unravel the spine, sending the tailbone away from you, bringing the pelvis back to neutral as you also lengthen the head and upper spine back to the starting neutral position.

5 Breathe in and hold the neutral position.

6 Breathe out and gently shine your chest forwards, collar-bones opening. This is a subtle movement, do not allow the lower back to dip, your pelvis stays neutral.

Repeat *up to 10 times, then come back into the Rest Position..*

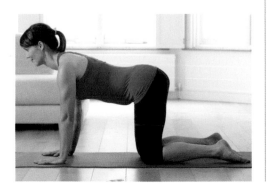

Variation **The Oblique Cat** This stretches your back and sides out beautifully. *Suitable for...* All stages. Later Pregnancy – in the last few weeks you may find your bump gets in the way, so stick with the normal Cat. Caution in the first few weeks Postnatal.

Starting position...

Four-point Kneeling. Before you start, practise one normal Cat as shown opposite. Place your left hand in front of your right hand. You are at an angle now, but try to stay lengthened through the waist.

Zip up to maintain a constant and appropriate connection to your centre throughout the exercise.

Action...

1 Breathe in to prepare your body, lengthen your spine.

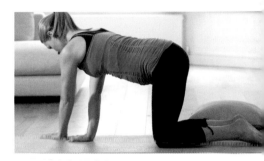

2 Breathe out as you roll your pelvis underneath you as for the Cat.

3 Breathe in wide to the lower ribcage to help maintain this lengthened C shape.

4 Breathe out as you unravel the spine, and come back to the starting neutral position.

Repeat *5 times, then repeat on the other side.*

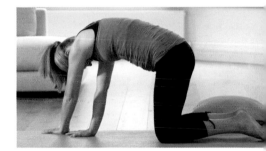

Oblique Rest option

You may come back to the Oblique Rest position after doing the exercise on one side, using whatever pillows you need and leaving your hands one in front of the other to achieve a gentle side stretch. After a few breaths, come back into Four-point Kneeling before doing Oblique Cat on the other side. Finish by either coming back into The Oblique Rest Position, then come back up into Four-point Kneeling; otherwise, roll back up centrally, restacking the vertebrae one by one.

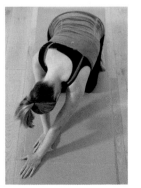

Seated Waist Twist

This simple but effective exercise will teach you how to rotate the spine sequentially with length and control. An added bonus is that it also works the muscles around your waist, which will be starting to disappear! With regular Pilates practice, you can look forward to it putting an early appearance back in after the birth. *Suitable for...* All stages.

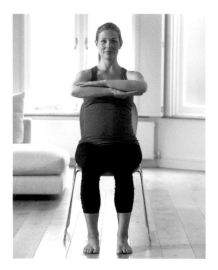

Starting position...

Seated on a chair. Fold your arms in front of your chest, just below shoulder height. One palm is on top of the opposite elbow and the other hand is positioned underneath the opposite elbow.

Zip up to maintain a constant and appropriate connection to your centre throughout the exercise.

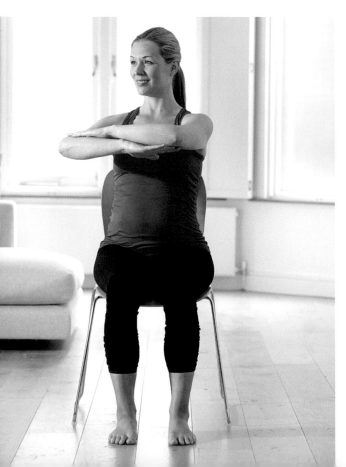

Action...

1 Breathe in to prepare to move, and lengthen your spine.

2 Breathe out as you turn first your head, then neck, then torso to the right. Keep your pelvis stable and keep lengthening up through the crown of the head.

3 Breathe in as you continue to lengthen your spine and rotate back, torso, neck and head to the Starting position.

Repeat *up to 5 times to each side.*

✳ Watchpoints

– Your pelvis should remain still. Keep the weight even on both sitting bones throughout.

– Keep both sides of your waist equally lengthened.

– Carry your arms with the spine; do not allow them to lead the movement.

– Think of spirally upwards both as you turn around and spirally upwards as you turn back to the centre.

Tennis Ball Rising

A mini squat which brings all the benefits of squatting (see page 153). This easy-to-do-anywhere exercise strengthens the ankles and feet, helps postural awareness and balance control. It also stretches the calves gently, so may help if you are getting leg cramps at night. *Suitable for...* All stages.

Starting position...

Stand tall on the floor sideways to a sturdy chair or a wall, which you may use for balance if you wish. Your legs are parallel and slightly closer than hip-width apart. If using a ball, place it between your ankles, just below the inside ankle bones.

Zip up to maintain a constant and appropriate connection to your centre throughout the exercise.

Action...

1 Breathe in to prepare your body and lengthen your spine.

2 Breathe out and rise up onto the balls of your feet, lifting your heels off the floor. Keep your spine lengthened and stable and maintain the position of the tennis ball (if using) in between your ankles.

3 Breathe in as you lower your heels back down to the floor, lengthening away from the crown of your head.

4 Breathe out as you softly bend your knees, keeping your heels on the floor.

5 Breathe in as you straighten your legs and return to the Starting position.

Repeat *up to 8 times.*

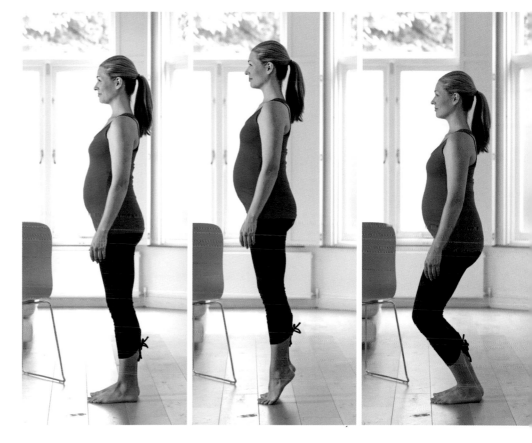

> **✳ Watchpoints**
> – Even when you are going down, think up, up and away.
> – Stay long in your waist.
> – Keep your weight balanced evenly on both feet.
> – Do not allow your feet to roll either in or out – if you do you may lose your tennis ball!
> – Maintain correct alignment of your legs; ensure that your ankles and knees remain in line with your hips.
> – Keep your chest and the front of your shoulders open and avoid any tension in your neck area.

Foot Exercises

Never have your feet been so important. A lot of foot problems start during pregnancy and many do not resolve themselves. The extra weight you are carrying puts enormous pressure on the arches and joints of the feet. These, in turn, are affected by the ligamentous laxity. The end result may be aching feet or, at worst, collapsed arches. The sooner you start the foot exercises the better and you should continue to do them right through your pregnancy and beyond. Exercises such as Tennis Ball Rising, Wall Slides, Pilates Squats will also help strengthen your feet.

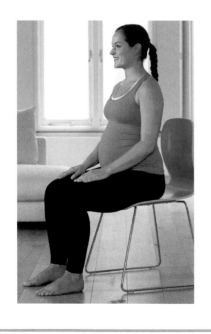

Working the Arches

This exercises targets the arches. It is a subtle movement which is easy to miss so please follow the directions carefully. *Suitable for...* All stages.

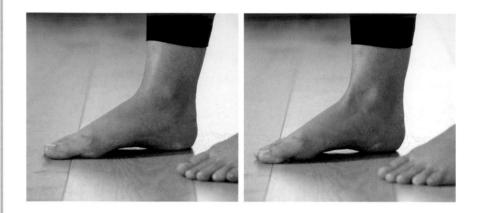

Starting position...

Sit upright on a chair so that the soles of your feet are on the floor. Have your legs hip-width apart and parallel. Relax your core muscles and breathe naturally throughout.

Action...

1 Keeping the toes long and not allowing them to scrunch up, draw the base of the toes back towards the heels thus increasing the arches.

2 Release the feet, returning to a lengthened position.

Repeat *up to 10 times, either working the feet separately or both together.*

✳ Watchpoints

– Avoid curling the toes; keep the action in the arches of the feet.

– Compare the action in this exercise to Creeping Toes, it should feel different.

– You may mimic the action with your hands if that helps.

– Ensure that the feet remain evenly planted on the floor and do not roll out or in.

– Maintain good hip, knee and ankle alignment.

– Imagine you are picking something up with the arch (not the toes) of the foot.

Mexican Wave

This one will keep you and any nearby children amused for hours. It is worth persevering with this exercise as it gently mobilises the joints in your feet. Notice that we are allowing a relaxation of the core muscles for this exercise. This will give you an all-important break when you do a session. *Suitable for...* All stages.

Starting position...

Sit upright on a chair, with your feet grounded hip-width apart on the floor. Relax your core muscles for this exercise and breathe naturally throughout.

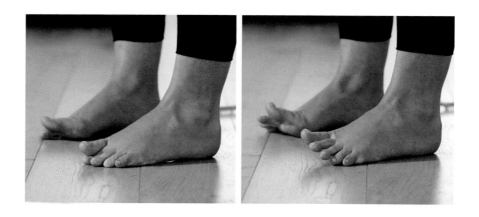

Action...

1   First, the warm up! Lift only your big toes off the floor, keeping the rest of your toes down.

2   Then, replace the big toes and try lifting all the others, leaving the big toe down.

3   Replace the toes.

4   Now try the full wave: try to lift the big toe then each and every toe off the floor one at a time in sequence until all of the toes have been peeled off. Check that you haven't cheated by rolling your foot in or out!

5   Replace your toes back down in sequence, starting with the little toe and spacing them out as wide as possible.

6   Reverse the movement: raise the little toes first, continuing one toe at a time to the big toe. (Note: achieving this may be a lifetime's work!)

Repeat *up to 5 times, either working the feet separately or both together.*

✳ Watchpoints

–   Ensure that your foot, ankle and knee remain in line with your hip.

–   If necessary, to begin with, use your hands to help guide the movement and isolate the toes. You will obviously have to sit down to do this.

–   Continue to maintain a stable and lengthened vertical position of your pelvis and spine throughout (unless you are using your hands to help).

Creeping Toes

This foot exercise strengthens and mobilises the arches and joints of the feet and the toes. *Suitable for...* All stages.

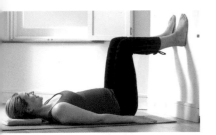

Starting position...
Lie on the mat facing a wall and place the feet up onto the wall. The entire soles of the feet are in contact with the wall. The knees and hip are flexed to approximately 90 degrees. The legs are hip-width and parallel. Core muscles can take a break! Breathe naturally throughout.

Later pregnancy option
Sit on a chair and creep the feet along the floor!

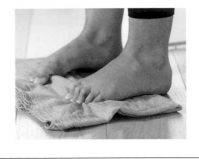

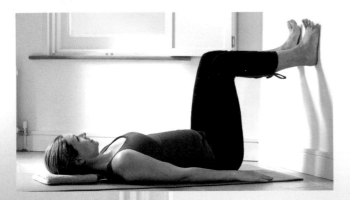

Action...
1 Spread the toes as wide as possible, and then scrunch them up so that they drag your feet a little up the wall. Maintain contact of the feet to the wall (or floor) throughout.

2 Repeat as above and continue creeping the feet up the wall until they can no longer stay flat.

3 Bend the knees and slide the feet back down the wall returning to the starting position.

Repeat *up to 5 times.*

✳ Watchpoints
– Ensure that the feet remain evenly planted on the wall or floor.
– Maintain good hip, knee and ankle alignment.

Ankle Circles

When you are pregnant your circulation suffers and by the end of the day your feet and ankles may look swollen. This easy exercise will help improve the circulation in your lower legs and will also mobilise your ankle joint. *Suitable for...* All stages.

Starting position...

The Relaxation Position. Fold one leg in towards your body with stability. If you wish, you may clasp your hands lightly behind your thigh and lift your lower leg up slightly so that your foot is higher than your knee.

Action...

1   Keeping your leg still, flex your foot towards you moving only your ankle joint and circle your foot outwards. Complete a full circle trying to keep your foot and toes lengthened and free from tension.

2   Repeat the ankle circle up to 5 times and then reverse the direction and circle the ankle up to 5 times inwards.

Repeat *on the other ankle, up to 5 times in each direction.*

Later pregnancy option

Sit tall in a chair. Ensure that your weight is still evenly distributed on both sitting bones. Reach down and support your working leg with your hands. As before you may now relax your core muscles and breathe naturally throughout.

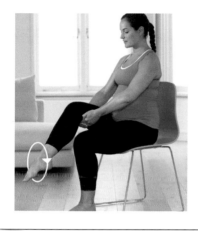

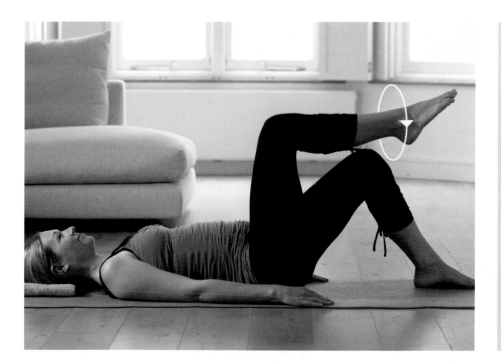

✳ Watchpoints

–   Keep your pelvis centred and grounded, taking care not to twist. This applies whether you are lying or sitting.

–   Keep your thigh and your shin bone still and correctly aligned throughout. Remember, you want the circle to come purely from your ankle.

–   Attempt to create full and even circles. You may notice a sticky bit but focus on trying to free this part of the circle.

–   Keep your chest and the front of your shoulders open and avoid any tension in your neck area.

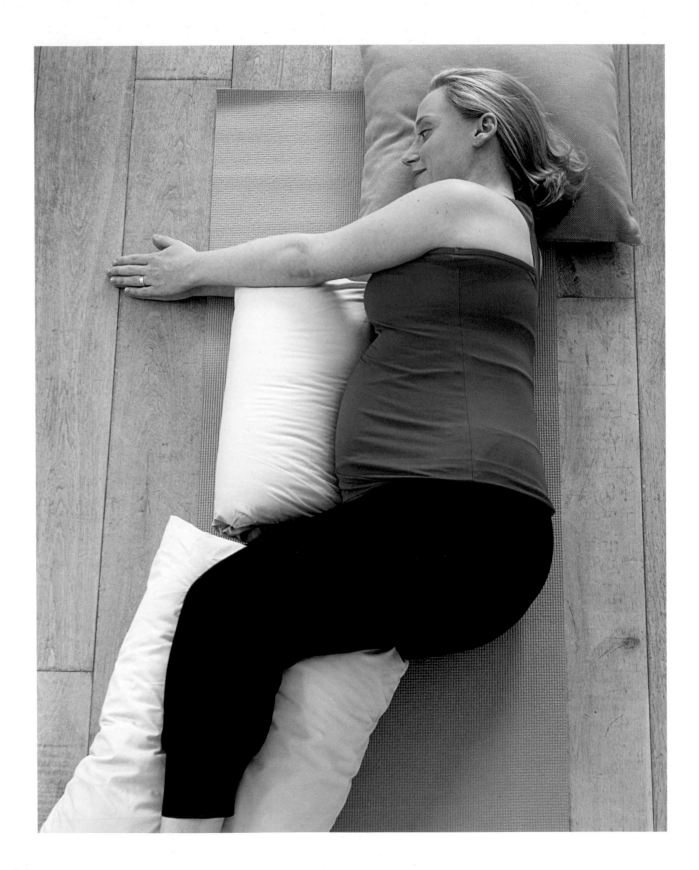

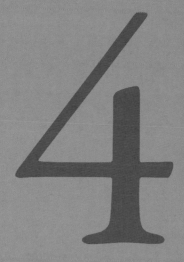

The Later Pregnancy Programme

The Later Pregnancy Programme

If you are joining the antenatal programme at this stage – welcome! We are going to take a few moments to take a look at your changing body so that you better understand your exercise needs at this time. We will then be asking you to go back and revise some other chapters in the book before you start but for now read on.

Some mothers continue to feel exhausted, especially if they have other young children to chase after or a heavy work schedule. If this applies to you, you still need to ensure that you plan your time carefully, maintaining that balance of work and play, being active and getting rest, that we discussed in the Early Pregnancy Programme.

Your changing body

By 16 weeks your baby's life support, the placenta, will be fully formed and your body should have grown more accustomed to being pregnant. The next few weeks are the time when most mothers feel really well, the queasiness has gone, your energy has returned. The pregnancy glow is not a myth – you only need to look at our models to see that mothers-to-be are often radiant. Of course there are exceptions to this rule.

Your growing bump and your abdominal muscles

The outside world will probably have noticed your condition now as your bump grows. By about 16 weeks the top of your uterus is nearly halfway to your navel, at 18 weeks it reaches your navel, and at 36 weeks it lies just below your diaphragm and starts competing with your ribs for space. One of our goals is to help create more space.

You may have noticed that your navel now protrudes. There will be changes in the pigmentation of your skin and the linea alba which runs from your navel down will darken in colour and becomes known as the linea nigra due to this darkening. Hollowing your lower abdominals back to your spine may sound like an impossible task! Obviously you are not going to get a hollow now! You will still be using The Wind Zip (page 60), but notice now that when you zip up and connect to your core, your bump gently lifts, as shown below.

It is as if you are hugging your baby. So visualise zipping up and hugging the baby as you connect to your core. Remember too the important role these core muscles play in supporting your bump and your back!

We noted on page 23 that your growing bump will also start to stretch and divide your abdominal muscles. With this in mind we are now going to avoid exercises which strongly use the abdominals, that is, Curl Up type exercises. Your practitioner should be keeping an eye on this divide. If this becomes very wide, your practitioner may advise you to not only avoid Curl Up type exercises, but also to take care with rotation and side flexion exercises, especially if they are strenuous. We have avoided this strenuous type of exercise in the book but if you are

uncertain which exercises are suitable for you, you can always take this book along with you to your check-ups and ask if any movements are contraindicated.

The good news is, however, that we have a hundred and one other ways of making you work those abdominals safely, which will hopefully mean that regaining your figure after the baby will be a lot easier.

Your digestion

We discussed in the opening chapters some of the more inconvenient conditions of pregnancy. You may experience heartburn, constipation, bloating and flatulence as your digestive system is sluggish. Bear in mind that gentle exercise can be very beneficial in helping to get things moving! But it is best to plan your Pilates practice so that you are not exercising after a meal. Eat something light perhaps a couple of hours before your session to sustain you. If you normally workout in the evening, you will not want to be eating a heavy meal after the session late in the evening or indigestion will keep you up all night! You may find that exercises such as Floating Arms and Ribcage Closure will help to take the pressure off the diaphragm and help with indigestion. Keeping good posture helps too!

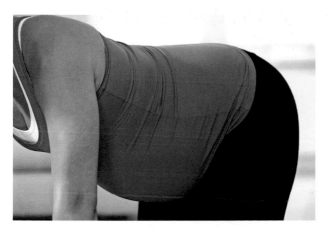

The Wind Zip

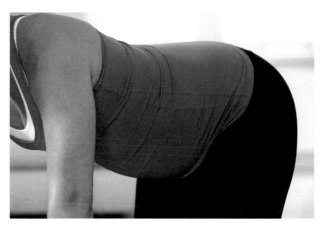

Supine Hypotensive Syndrome

This condition, which may affect you from about 16 weeks onwards, is going to have an impact on the type of exercises you do in this Later Pregnancy Programme. Let's look first at exactly what it is, then we can work out how to avoid it.

Supine means lying flat on your back. (Semi-supine is lying flat with the knees bent, that is Relaxation Position). Hypotension is low blood pressure.

Thus, supine hypotensive syndrome is low blood pressure brought on by lying flat. Supine hypotensive syndrome can happen if you are lying flat on your back and the pressure from the uterus and baby can block the vena cava, the largest vein in the trunk, and restrict blood flow to the heart. If this happens you may feel faint or nauseous. Not all women feel this, some women report that they feel fine lying on their back, but it makes sense to avoid lying in any position which may interrupt the blood flow to the baby.

Most women instinctively roll over if they feel dizzy. When you do move, the symptoms should disappear quickly. In a normal Pilates workout there are a lot of exercises which involve lying on your back. We need to change this for you. In fact, you may have already noticed when looking at the exercises in The Fundamentals, Preparing for Pregnancy and Early Pregnancy programmes that we have suggested alternative Starting positions, where possible, avoiding supine and semi-supine, for Later Pregnancy.

There are other options, for example placing a pillow under the right side of the body. This tips the trunk to avoid the problem but interferes with your alignment. The other alternative is to raise the head and shoulders 20–30 degrees with pillows or wedges. These might be suitable for some exercises but, for simplicity, we have avoided exercises lying on your back at this stage.

Even though we are going to avoid lying flat, you should still stay alert to any signs of hypotension (see below) and roll onto your left side if you feel dizzy. Remember this may affect you at other times, for example in bed or if you have a massage.

Standing still for too long can make your blood

Supine Hypotensive Syndrome

Signs of Supine Hypotensive Syndrome	Nausea and vomiting
Pallor	Chest and abdominal discomfort
Muscle twitching	Visual disturbances
Shortness of breath	Numbness of limbs
Yawning	Headache
Cold, clammy skin	Cold legs
A wild expression	Weakness
	Tinnitus
Symptoms	Fatigue
Faintness	Desire to flex hips and knees
Dizziness	
Restlessness	Anguish

pressure drop too, so if you are doing a standing exercise only perform a few repetitions. If you are stuck standing on the train or in a queue, try Walking on the Spot (page 161), it may just help get the blood circulating again until you can move or sit down.

Posture Check

We saw in the opening chapters that your centre of gravity is going to alter as your uterus and baby grow. If you have not already done so, now is the time to check your posture or ask a friend to help. You can use the Posture Assessment on page 34. Remember that your posture will be changing month by month so do recheck regularly. Take note again of whether you have an increased lumbar curve (Posture A) or a decreased lumbar curve (Posture B). Either way, we want you to find that comfortable mid-neutral position. Include the appropriate Wall Slides to help remind you where this is, then try to take awareness of this when you sit and stand. You may find that you carry your weight more through your heels, rather than your arches. Once again try to be aware if this is happening and remember all the good standing directions we gave you on page 53.

Meanwhile your breasts will be growing substantially. By the end of your pregnancy they may have increased their weight by as much as 900g. Do invest in a good supportive non-wired bra. You are going to need good mid-back muscles to keep your upper body in good alignment and to carry the weight of the breasts. Normally we would target these muscles and help encourage your upper back to extend (bend backwards) by using exercises where you lie on your front. This may be an option for a while, but it will soon become too uncomfortable and you should avoid lying prone after 20 weeks. We have used different positions to help your upper body posture. You will notice lots of gentle rotation exercises in the programme; these will help keep your upper spine mobile.

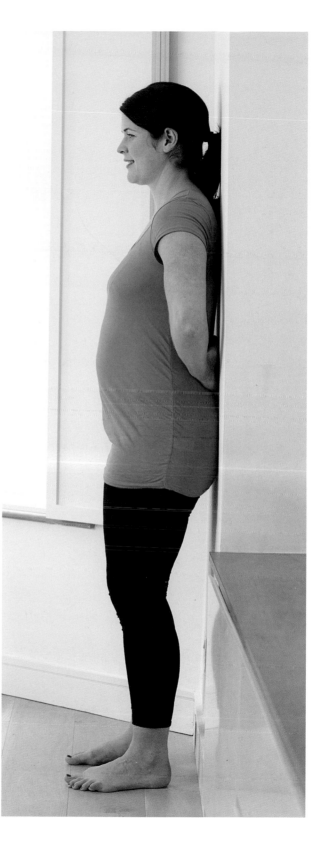

Your joints

We have discussed at length the effect of ligamentous laxity on all your joints (page 17). With this in mind we will continue to work on toning the muscles that support your joints, while avoiding any movements that may place any strain on them. In particular, we will avoid any movements that may put a strain on your sacroiliac joints and your symphysis pubis joint. For the same reason, we will avoid overstretching the hamstring (back of thigh) and adductor (inner thigh) muscles. However, we have to achieve a balance here. The last thing you need are tight inner thigh muscles for the birth! Gentle dynamic stretches where the stretch to both sides is even is the answer. A lot of the seated Starting positions on the mat and by the wall will help to gently stretch out your thighs. Zig Zags and Squats with the legs apart turned out from the hip joints and will also help.

Common conditions

In the first chapter we mentioned how hormonal changes are going to cause the relaxation of the muscle tissue in your veins; this combined with an increase in blood volume and fluid retention means that you may suffer from mild swelling of the lower legs. For the same reasons you are also more likely to get piles and varicose veins. Veins carry blood from the extremities back to the heart. To do this they have to work against gravity so to help them they have a series of valves that prevent the backflow of blood. Unfortunately if the valves are not working well, blood can pool in the veins, especially in the legs and the rectum. This results in a bulging of the veins – that is varicose veins and haemorrhoids. The extra weight gain of pregnancy, the relaxation of the muscle tissue, the increase in blood volume and the added pressure of the uterus on the pelvic area all compound the problem.

Fortunately, there are lots of Pilates exercises which boost the circulatory and lymphatic systems and help to keep those fluids moving. Exercises such as Walking on the Spot and Tennis Ball Rising work the deep calf pump and help the valves to work efficiently. Ankle Circles help too. Pelvic floor exercises (we have included plenty of these) will improve circulation to the pelvic area. You can also help by not standing for too long, wearing support tights and socks, avoiding high heels, drinking plenty of water to avoid constipation and thus avoiding straining, and by keeping your weight gain within

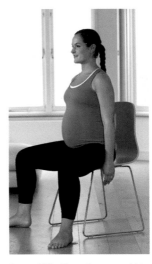

Seated Zig Zags *See page 164*

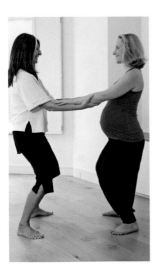

Partner Squats *See pages 174–175*

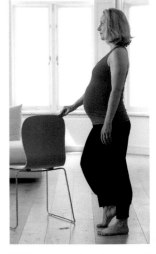

Walking on the Spot *See page 161*

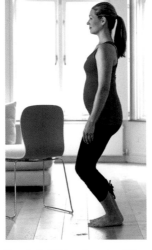

Tennis Ball Rising *See page 127*

'Before any real benefit can be derived from physical exercises, one must first learn how to breathe properly. Our very life depends on it.'

Joseph Pilates

guidelines. Simply going for walk will also help to get the calf pump working.

You may find that fluid accumulation can result in leg cramps. These can happen at any time but are most likely at night after the fluids have collected in the legs all day. We have shown you a Calf Stretch to help (page 162). Try to avoid standing for long periods. Make sure that you do not do too many standing exercises in a row. Occasionally pointing the toes can also cause a leg cramp. If you do get one – the key is to flex the foot bringing the toes down towards your face. Otherwise, you can help to prevent them by elevating the legs during the day.

Breathing

As your pregnancy progresses you will experience respiratory changes mainly due to fluid retention and the simple fact that the uterus is pushing up on the diaphragm and causing the lower ribs to lift and flare. You may find yourself short of breath. Remember, do not panic, it does not mean that either you or the baby will be short of oxygen. The changes actually allow you to take in more oxygen. You may feel as though you need to breathe more deeply. The lateral thoracic breathing that you have been practising in Pilates will help you here. So will good posture. Slouching will only close the ribcage down and restrict your breathing so stand and sit tall. You may find that you have to alter the breathing from the directions given in the exercises. This is fine. The main thing to remember is not to over-breathe or you may make yourself dizzy, and never ever hold your breath while exercising.

Taking a few quiet moments to focus on your breathing and your baby will prove very beneficial. In the chapter on Preparing for Labour and the Birth we will also explore some breathing techniques to help during labour.

Braxton Hicks

From about your 20th week, your uterus has been rehearsing for the birth itself with practice contractions, known as Braxton Hicks. These are simply warm-ups for the birth. As you approach your due date, these contractions can become strong enough to require you to take time out and rest. You may find it difficult to concentrate while the uterus flexes its own muscles. If you are comfortable, it would be the perfect opportunity to practice Relaxation techniques until they pass. If they haven't stopped after 30 minutes then seek medical advice, you might be in labour! Rarely, the action of zipping up and connecting to your core can set the Braxton Hicks off. If this is the case, then you will have to stop the session and try again later.

Nearly there

As your due date approaches and you become heavier and more restricted in your movements, it becomes even more important for you to practise Pilates. You may not feel as graceful, but there are enormous benefits to be had from exercising right up to the end as long as you are feeling well, are pain free and have continued medical clearance. There are so many ways in which exercise can help prepare you for the birth. See the chapter on Preparation for the Birth.

If this is your first child, then about 2–4 weeks before the birth, the baby's head may engage. This is known as the lightening, and occurs when the presenting part of the baby (hopefully the head!) drops into the upper bony part of the pelvis in readiness for the birth. It doesn't always happen before labour and with second and subsequent pregnancies it usually happens during labour itself rather than before. As the baby's head engages there is less pressure on the ribcage – making breathing easier. The bad news is that there is now more pressure on the pelvic floor. Try not to waddle if you can help it!

We have been advocating plenty of rest throughout the book and it continues to be extremely important to balance rest and activity. Your blood pressure will be closely monitored by your antenatal clinic during this trimester, as it can rise during this period. High blood pressure is a symptom of pre-eclampsia, which affects 5–10 per cent of pregnant women and, if left unchecked, it can lead to eclampsia – a very serious condition for both mother and baby. To help keep your stress levels low make sure that your workouts include plenty of relaxation exercises. If you are resting try to lie on your left side.

A few gentle exercises before you go to bed may help still your mind and help you sleep. You are going to need lots of 'me' time, time to put your feet up but you must also stay active and fit in preparation for the hard work of labour and motherhood! Do not leave reading the chapter on Preparing for the Birth until the day before you are due. You are going to need time to practise the movements, positions, breathing and pelvic floor control exercises.

Now, if you have been following the Early Pregnancy Programme, you may turn to page 148 for Exercise Guidelines for Later Pregnancy, the Later Pregnancy exercises and Preparing for Labour. Of course, you may also refresh your memory of The Fundamentals.

If you are joining us here, that is, if you are new to this Pilates programme, we are going to introduce you to the Fundamentals of Pilates before you start the Later Pregnancy exercises. You will find these on page 150.

Commonly asked questions

Question: **I'm finding it really hard to release my pelvic floor and I'm worried about the delivery, is there anything I can do?**
A healthy pelvic floor is essential for pregnancy and the birthing process. The pelvic floor muscle can be tight or overactive for many reasons, such as habitual sitting with legs crossed. Tension in the pelvic floor can compress the bladder causing discomfort and urgency, and more relevantly, can lengthen the labour phase. Thus it is important to gain control over these muscles.

Pelvic floor exercises encourage the soft tissues to be more elastic and well toned, and most importantly, stretch more easily. It is important to develop awareness of how to gently contract and fully relax the pelvic floor muscles. Release of the pelvic floor muscles can be achieved through breathing and relaxation exercises and specific release exercises such as those on page 108.

If you are aware of a specific problem, or have concerns that you are still not able to release your pelvic floor, your midwife or GP may be able to offer advice, or refer you to an obstetric (women's health) physiotherapist.

There is also some excellent advice on pelvic floor release online – see the physiotherapy websites listed in Further Information, page 223.

Question: **Since I've been pregnant I've been getting pins and needles in my hands when I wake up. What can I do?**
Pins and needle in the hands during pregnancy may be caused by compression of one of the main nerves that travel into the hand, through a bony space in the wrist called the carpal tunnel.

The condition is called carpal tunnel syndrome, and commonly occurs in the second and third trimesters, as the onset is caused by swelling resulting from the increased fluid retention and weight gain experienced naturally during pregnancy.

The symptoms include pins and needles, numbness and pain in the thumb, first and middle fingers, and half of the fourth finger, and can progress to pain in the wrist, hand and forearm. The symptoms are typically worse at night, as gravity causes the fluids to collect in the hands during the day, resulting in increased swelling and pressure.

The problem may be alleviated by wearing splints (see Further Information, page 223) to keep the wrists in a neutral position and allow greater space for the nerve tissues. This is especially important at night, to avoid the tendency to sleep on the hands or tuck them up excessively.

Being aware of good upper body posture and movement patterns may be helpful. Try the following exercises as long they feel comfortable: Floating Arms, Ribcage Closure, Dumb Waiter and Variations, Chest Expansion. Care is required when exercising as you need to keep a neutral alignment of the hand, wrist and shoulder. During Four-point Kneeling, try using a rolled up towel under the hands, or a folded towel or flat cushion under the heels of the hands to reduce the angle of the wrist as on page 47. Alternatively try resting the forearms on a chair.

The symptoms usually resolve soon after the birth of the baby, but if the symptoms persist, the GP may refer you for physiotherapy treatment.

Question: **I'm 30 weeks pregnant and over the last few weeks I've had bad heel pain. Is there anything I can do?** Pain in the heels during pregnancy may be caused by damage to the long fibrous plantar fascia ligament that runs along the bottom of the foot from the heel bone to the forefoot.

The natural weight gain during pregnancy alters the centre of gravity, and this, combined with the hormonal changes that cause the ligament to soften, may exert extra pressure through the soft tissues, leading to pain and swelling, typically at the point where the ligament attaches to the heel bone. Take special note of standing well with your weight centered over your arches.

The symptoms often resolve with a combination of a change of activity, rest, ice and the use of more supportive footwear or simple orthotic devices that reduce the loading and allow healing to occur. The following foot exercises may prove helpful as long as they do not increase your pain: Wall Slides, Calf stretching, Ankle circles, Zig Zags and Creeping Toes. If however, the symptoms persist after the baby is born, it is important to seek medical advice to avoid the problem becoming chronic. The GP may refer you to a physiotherapist or podiatrist for further management.

For more information visit www.plantar-fasciitis.org

Good Posture in Your Daily Activities

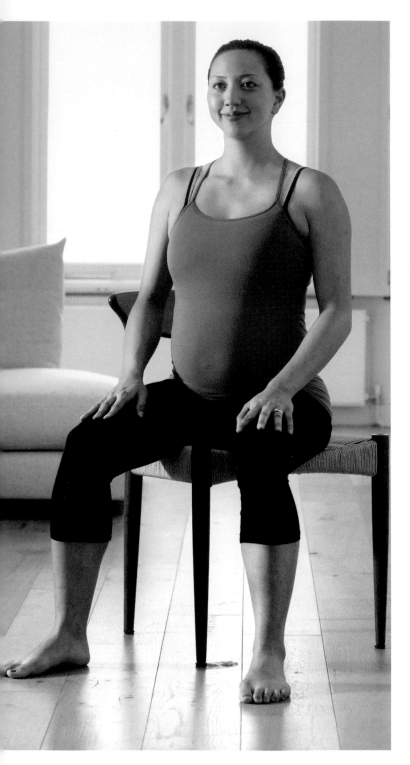

If at a desk

The single most important thing to remember when seated is to keep the natural 'S curve' of the spine (see page 33). Do not allow yourself to sink back into a slumped 'C curve'.

Chairs or sofas that are too soft, too low or too deep will not encourage you to sit well. Initially they might feel relaxing, but this is short-lived.

If you happen to be seated on a chair with a square base and no arms, try turning the chair at an angle and sitting on the corner. You should find it opens the hips. Your feet will be wider than hip-width in this case.

Sitting well at your desk *Regardless of the type of chair, the following instructions should help.*

✷ Sit on your sitting bones. You can feel these when you sit on a hard chair and place your hands under each buttock. By transferring your weight from cheek to cheek, you can feel the sitting bones. The weight should be evenly distributed between those bones. Try to keep your pelvis in neutral.

✷ Your feet should be planted firmly on the floor, hip-width apart. If your feet do not easily reach the floor then place them on a footstool or telephone directory.

✷ When sitting on normal chairs where the seat is parallel to the floor try to keep the lower part of your legs at 90 degrees to the thighs. The height of the chair is, therefore, very important. If it is too high your feet will be dangling – in this case, a footstool as mentioned above can help. If the seat is too low (a problem with some sofas) you are increasing the pressure on the lower back, as it is much harder to maintain the natural curves of the spine.

✱ The back of your knee to the seat edge should be 5cm so as not to restrict blood circulation to the lower leg.

✱ Avoid crossing your legs, as this will twist your spine and restrict circulation in the legs.

✱ Keep your back long with its natural 'S curve' still present. When you are slouching you are making a collapsed 'C curve' and are, therefore, increasing the pressure on joints and discs.

✱ Try not to perch too far forward on the edge of the chair.

✱ Supporting the lower (lumbar) back is sometimes necessary, especially if your core stabilising muscles are not yet strong enough to do the job. A good chair provides this, but a lumbar roll or a small cushion can equally be as effective.

✱ Relax your shoulders and thighs.

✱ Avoid sitting for long periods of time. Move about every half an hour to stretch the back and decrease the pressure.

✱ The position of your head is very important. It is very heavy and can pull the spine out of alignment. Keep your neck soft and tension free.

✱ The height of the desk is as important as the height of the chair. To determine the right height, bear in mind that, when working on a personal computer, your forearms and wrists should be parallel or slightly sloping downwards from the desk.

✱ The height of the screen is also crucial. The centre of the screen should be level with your eyes, so that you are not tipping your head back or down. Propping the screen up with the help of books can be useful.

✱ You should not need to strain to read the screen, if necessary, work with a larger font size.

✱ Legs should be under the desk, so that you do not have to reach forward to the keyboard. The desk should therefore be quite deep.

✱ Avoid cradling the telephone in your neck! Keep both shoulder-blades down and your neck released. If you are a heavy telephone user, use a headset or, if circumstances allow, a hands-free telephone.

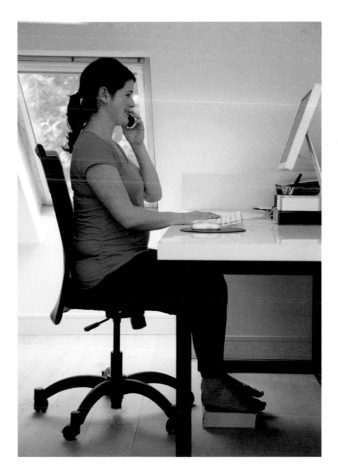

Getting up from a chair

When you get up from a chair, place your feet hip-width apart, but with one foot in front of the other. Hinge as you lean forward over your legs and keeping the natural curves in your back (not allowing the back to overarch or over hollow) lengthen through the top of the head and rise up using your thigh and back muscles.

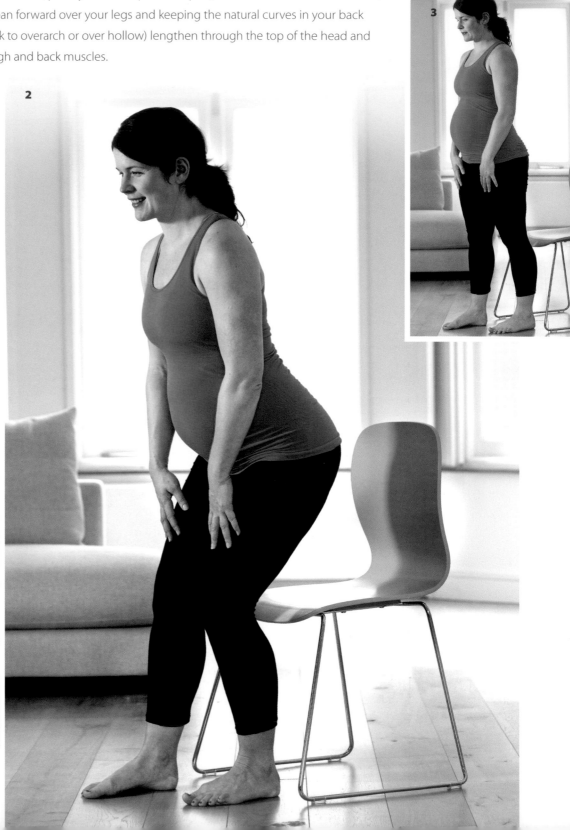

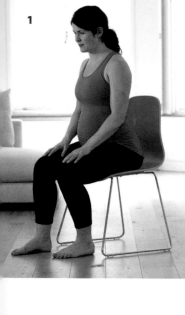

Sleeping well

A good night's rest is vital to us all, pregnant or not pregnant! It is while you sleep, that a lot of the body's repair work at cellular level takes place, and the body therefore regenerates itself.

* The choice of bed is important. It should be supportive and comfortable. If the mattress is too soft, your back will not be supported, and if it is too hard it does not give at your shoulders and hips. You will therefore lose the natural curves of your spine.

* The bigger the bed the more space you have to move around, and you are less likely to sleep in one awkward position.

* If at all possible try to sleep lying on your left side, with a collection of pillows to support you in this position.

* A pillow between your knees in particular can make you more comfortable.

Lifting and carrying well

It is inevitable that during your pregnancy you will still have to lift and carry either young children or heavy shopping. You should do your best to avoid lifting very heavy objects but if you *do* have to lift something heavy follow the advice given below and do not twist! Bear in mind that you will not have these guidelines with you at the time, so you need to practise the movements now.

* Where possible take the time to divide the load up. It may take a little longer to complete the task, but it is better than harming your back.

* Do not be afraid to ask someone to help you. An extra pair of hands will lighten the load.

* When you are about to lift something, it is important to position yourself correctly to start with.

* You should be aware of the weight of the object that you are about to lift.

* Stand as close as possible to the load and have your feet on either side of the load, with one foot slightly in front of the other, just as if you were taking a step.

* Bend at the knee and hip to bend down like a squat.

* Keep your back long and strongly supported by your core.

* Keeping your body close to the load, using the handles if available or placing one hand under the object with the other hand on top.

* As you lift, make sure you keep the load close to your body. The further away that you hold the load, the more you are straining your back.

* Lean forward and, while maintaining a long back, straighten your knees and hips.

* Avoid lifting and twisting at the same time. Lift first and then rotate the whole trunk round to where you want to go.

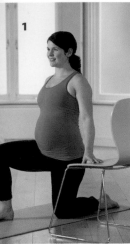

Getting onto the floor in later pregnancy and for up to six weeks after the birth

Slowly lower yourself onto one knee.

Then come onto both knees.

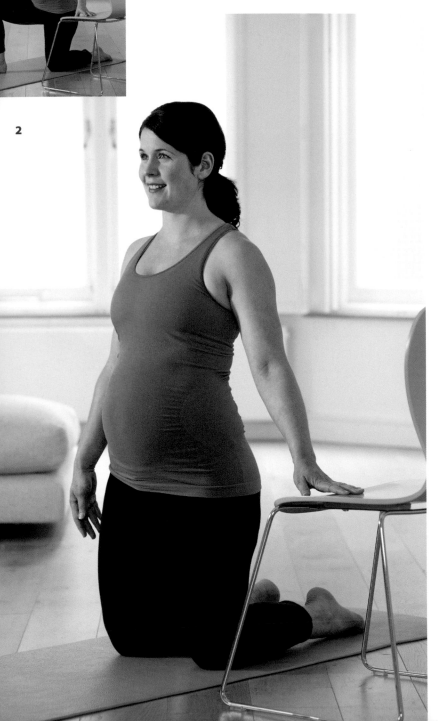

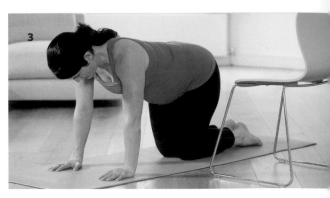

Place both hands onto the floor in front of you in a Four-point Kneeling position.

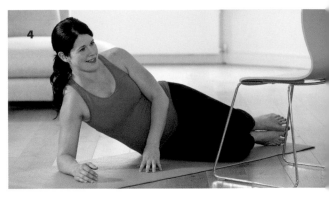

Then carefully move so that you are sitting to one side.

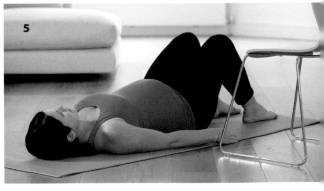

Now, zipping up and connecting to your core, bring your legs in front of you. Very slowly and with control lower yourself back USING YOUR ELBOWS. But remember not to lie on your back for more than a few moments.

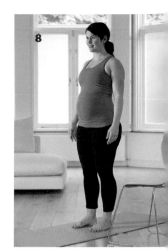

To come back up, you will reverse the actions. Roll onto your side keeping your knees bent. Use your hands to push yourself into a side-sitting position.

Then come onto all fours again. Bring one knee in front.

With your hand on your knee, push yourself into a standing position.

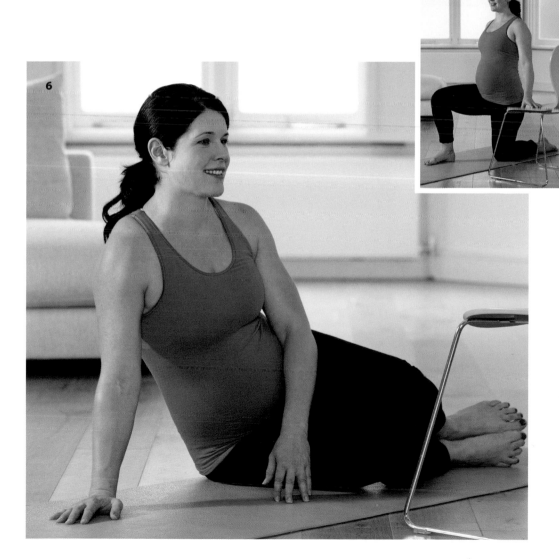

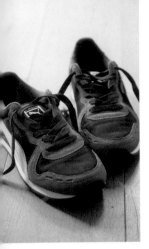

Clothing and footwear

Avoid tight clothing as it may restrict your circulation. Good supportive underwear is essential as your pregnancy progresses. Avoid underwired bras. Avoid the regular wearing of high heels while you are pregnant. They tend to throw the pelvis forward. Save them for special occasions. On the other hand, totally flat shoes, for example flip flops or ballet pumps, are equally a problem as they do not offer any support for your arches.

Exercise guidelines

Keep an array of pillows and cushions on hand as you exercise. But as it will become increasingly difficult for you to see your feet, make sure that the area where you are working is clear. Your pregnancy hormones can affect your spatial awareness, so take extra care especially if you are using any weights or equipment.

✳ Do not exercise if you feel tired. If you feel tired while exercising, stop and rest. Short sessions are still valuable.

✳ Avoid doing too many repetitions. Our directions say 'up to' so you don't have to complete them all.

✳ Change position slowly and frequently.

✳ Plan your sessions to take into account meal times and any indigestion you may suffer.

✳ Try not to do too many standing positions in a row.

✳ If you feel at all dizzy then lie on your left side – this is also an ideal position for resting.

✳ Think now of zipping up and lifting the bump, to help with your core connection.

✳ Take a moment to relax between exercises so that your abdominals can have a break.

✳ Avoid overstretching.

✳ If you want to stretch the hamstring (back of thigh) or adductor (inner thigh) muscles do so gently and evenly.

✳ You might like to use a wedge or a rolled up towel under the sitting bones when seated on a mat.

✳ Change the timing of the breathing if you are short of breath. Never hold your breath.

✳ Don't forget to do your foot exercises!

✳ Your pelvic floor work should now include lots and lots of release work, e.g. the Flower or the Elevator going down to basement to prepare for birth.

✳ Empty your bladder before a workout to save you having to interrupt the session and to avoid mishaps.

✳ Four-point Kneeling exercises will feel wonderful as they take the weight of the baby off the spine. If you have carpal tunnel syndrome, see page 40.

Air embolism

There is one thing that should be mentioned even though the chances of it happening are very, very remote. There have only ever been a few cases worldwide.

It can happen that with certain movements air is drawn into the vagina. Normally this is no problem (except perhaps for the embarrassing noise it can make!) but in a pregnant woman there is a risk of an air embolism occurring as the pressure change causes air to be sucked into the vagina and the uterus, where it can enter the circulatory system through the open placenta wound. There is particular danger if there is any bleeding or other symptoms of early placental displacement. There is more risk in the six weeks after the birth. Basically, you should avoid movements or positions which force air into the vagina, e.g. coming up quickly from a position where the head has been down and the buttocks are elevated, drawing the knee to the chest in Four-point Kneeling, or any position where the buttocks are elevated and the uterus moves upwards. We have deliberately avoided such movements in this book, but if you are also including other fitness techniques in your schedule, you must be aware of the potential dangers of such movements.

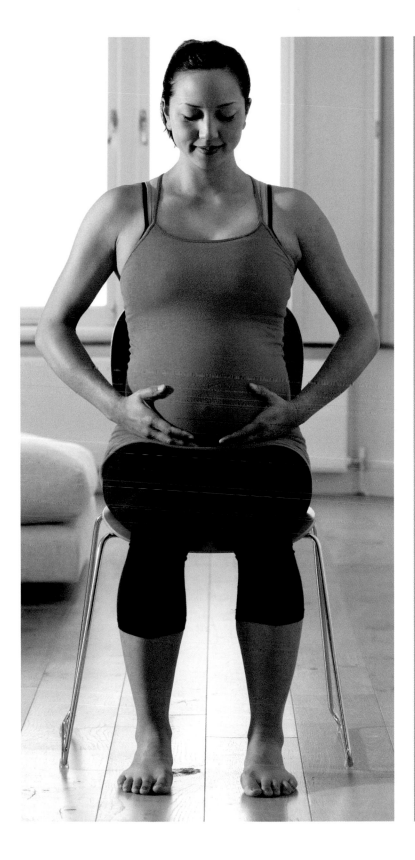

New to Pilates?

This little section of the programme has been written for those of you who are new to Pilates and are at least 16 weeks through your pregnancy. Remember that we do not advise you to take up Pilates for the first time before 16 weeks. Or perhaps you have done some Pilates but preferred, or were advised, to wait until 16 weeks before continuing.

Our Fundamental ABCs – Alignment, Breathing and Centring are the same no matter which stage of pregnancy you are in and apply to everyone doing Pilates. What will change, however, are the positions in which you can learn these Fundamentals.

Go back now and read through the whole of The Fundamentals chapter. As you read through the practice exercises you will notice that we have given you guidelines on which exercises are suitable for which stages of pregnancy.

Then practise the exercises on the following page, taking care to use the recommended Later Pregnancy positions:

The Fundamentals for Later Pregnancy

Alignment

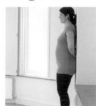

Posture Check
Page 137

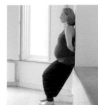

Wall Slides A or B
Page 36–39

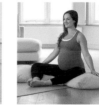

Seated on chair
Page 45

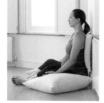

Seated on mat
Page 44

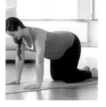

Seated by wall
cushions *Page 44*

Four-point Kneeling
Page 61

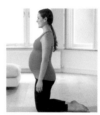

High Kneeling
Page 48

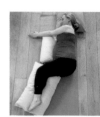

Side-lying (cushions)
Page 50

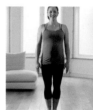

Standing Tall
Page 53

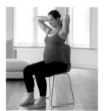

Pilates Stance
Page 52

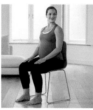

Neck Rolls and Chin Tucks
Page 54

Breathing

Scarf Breathing
Page 56

Centring

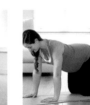

Wind Zip (seated)
Page 60

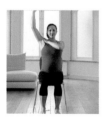

Four-point Kneeling
Page 61

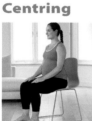

Floating Arms
Page 66

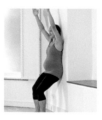

Ribcage Closure in
Wall Slide *Page 69*

You will also be able to include the following exercises from earlier in the book providing you only attempt the Later Pregnancy positions.

From the Preparing for Pregnancy Programme:

– Hip Rolls (do not rest in the Relaxation Position but keep moving keep a watch for supine hypotensive syndrome) *page 93*

– Shoulder Drops (seated with stretch band) *page 80*

– Table Top (keep the hands and feet in contact with the mat) *pages 96–97*

– Rest Position (with pillows) *page 98*

– Side Reach *(page 100)*

– Pelvic Floor Control *(page 104)*

From the Early Pregnancy Programme:

– Knee Rolls (seated on chair) *page 116*

– Cat (you will be limited a bit by the bump) *page 124*

– Seated Waist Twist *(page 126)*

– Tennis Ball Rising *(page 127)*

– Foot exercises *(pages 128–131)*

Later Pregnancy Workouts

Hopefully you will create your own workouts. Sit quietly and simply breathe and connect to your body. See if you can sense which movements your body would like to do… If possible try to include some spinal flexion, rotation, side flexion and extension. Pelvic Floor Control, Foot exercises and Preparation for Labour exercises. Here are two sample workouts to inspire you:

Workout One

Wall Slides A or B . . . . (pages 36–39)
Ribcage Closure in Wall Slide . . . . (page 69)
Seated Zig Zags . . . . page 164)
Seated Side Reach . . . . (page 100)
Seated Chest Extension . . . . (page 156)
Seated Scapular Squeeze . . . . (page 158)
Ankle Circles . . . . (page 131)
Pelvic Rocking . . . . (page 180)
Rest Position . . . . (page 98)
Side-lying Circles . . . . (page 166)
Arm Openings . . . . (page 160)
Pelvic Floor Control including release (seated on mat
   or by wall): . . . . (page 104)
Tennis Ball Rising . . . . (page 127)
Pilates Squat . . . . (page 153)

Workout   Two

Walking on the Spot . . . . (page 161)
Floating Arms . . . . (page 66)
Knee Rolls (seated on chair) . . . . (page 116)
Dumb Waiter . . . . (page 157)
Hip Hinge . . . . (page 152)
Working the Arches . . . . (page 128)
Mexican Wave . . . . (page 129)
Chest Expansion plus Rotation (High Kneeling) . (page 155)
Pelvic Rocking . . . . (page 180)
Tail Swish . . . . (page 182)
Rest Position . . . . (page 98)
Oyster . . . . (page 161)
Arm Openings . . . . (page 160)
Wrist Circles (seated on mat) . . . . (page 159)
Side Reach . . . . (page 100)
Seated Waist Twist . . . . (page 126)
Breathing and the Pelvic Floor (seated by wall) (page 108)
Pilates Squats . . . . (page 152)
Wall Slides A or B . . . . (pages 36–39)

Hip Hinge and Pilates Squats

The Pilates Squat is an all-round winner. Not only does it help to open your pelvic outlet in readiness for the birth, but it also helps to strengthen your thigh muscles, teaches correct alignment of the legs, mobilises and strengthens the hip and knee joints and challenges your core stability! It will also help to stretch the perineal area for flexibility during the labour itself. It gives you strength and endurance in the muscles needed for squatting during birth. To help perfect your squatting technique, practise The Hip Hinge first.

Hip Hinge *Suitable for...* All stages. The Pilates squat is a 'hip hinge' movement, we want the movement to come from the hips, not the spine, which should stay lengthened and move as one unit. Sounds strange but imagine that you have swallowed a long stick!

Starting position...

Sit on a sturdy chair, feet hip-width apart and parallel. You will need to be nearer the edge than the back of the chair. Press your hands palms down in the crease where your legs meet your pelvis.

Action...

1 Keeping the spine straight (but with its natural curves), hinge forward from this crease. The spine moves as one long unit.

2 Return to upright. Practise a few times before trying the Pilates Squat.

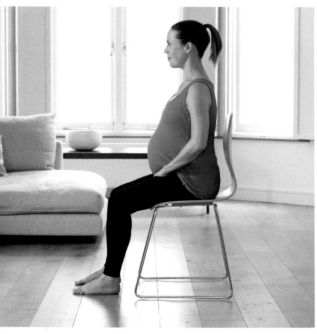

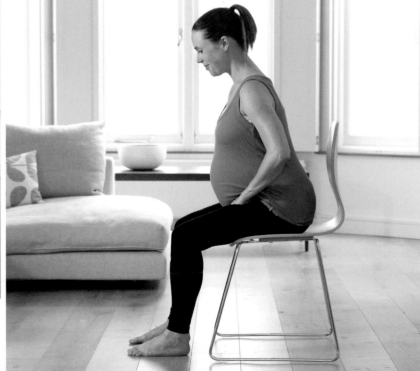

Pilates Squat *Suitable for...* All stages. However from 35 weeks, check with your midwife because if your baby is breech presentation, she may advise you to avoid squats for a while.

Starting position...
Initially, practise this standing sideways to a wall or sturdy chair, in case you lose your balance. Once again imagine you have swallowed a long stick. Stand tall. Arms relaxed down by your side, palms facing inwards.
Zip up to maintain a constant and appropriate connection to your centre throughout.

1 Breathe in to prepare the body, lengthen through the spine as you bend the knees and the hips simultaneously to hinge forwards slightly from the hips. As you do so, reach forwards with both arms, it will help to counter your balance.
2 Breathe out as you straighten the legs and return to the upright starting position.
Repeat *up to 10 times.*

Variation
Try this exercise holding light weights.

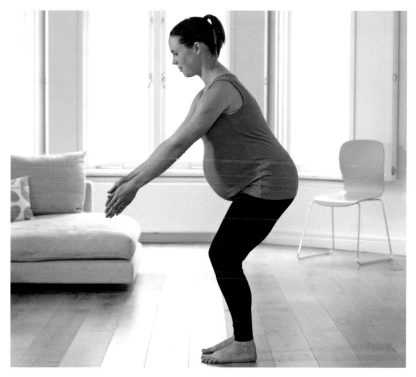

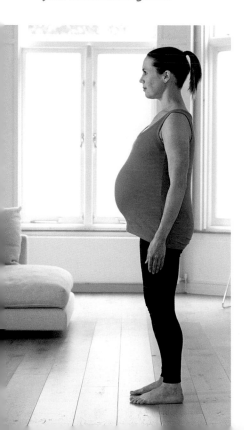

> **✳ Watchpoints**
> – Take care not to tip your head back. The back of the neck remains lengthened.
> – This is a small squat so do not go down too far, avoid lowering the pelvis below knee level.
> – Check that your ankles, knees and hips are lined up as you hinge forward.
> – Do not to allow your knees or ankles to buckle in or out.
> – As you straighten up, press the floor away evenly through the soles of the feet.
> – Keep the heels in contact with the floor throughout.
> – Sense the spine lengthening up and away.

Chest Expansion

This exercise is a great chest opener. It also helps your breathing technique. *Suitable for...* All stages. **Equipment** Optional hand-held weights up to 0.5kg per weight.

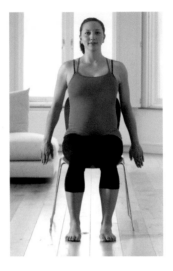 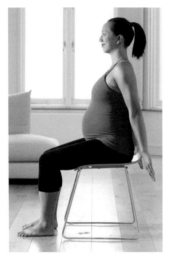 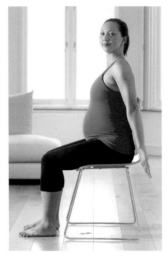 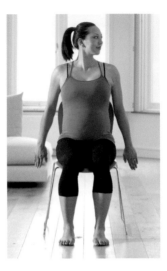

Starting position...

Sit on a chair, Stand Tall, or High Kneel. Hold the weights (if using) lengthening your arms down by the sides of your body with your palms facing backwards, just slightly in front of you. **Zip up to maintain a constant and appropriate connection to your centre throughout.**

Action...

1 Breathe in as you press your arms behind you as far as is possible without disturbing the position of your spine.

2 Still breathing in, turn your head to the left, then pass through the centre, and turn to the right.

3 Breathe out as you return your head to the centre and then lengthen the arms forward returning them slightly in front of the body. **Repeat** *up to 10 times, alternating the side of the first head turn each time.*

> **✳ Watchpoints**
> – Think of the exercise name – Chest Expansion. Breathe in to allow your chest to fully expand but take care not to arch your back or flare your ribs.
> – Move the arms only from the shoulder joints.
> – Turn your head on a central axis, not tipping it back or forwards.
> – Keep your hands and wrists in line with your forearm.
> – Keep your chest and the front of your shoulders open especially as you raise your arms forwards.
> – Release your neck and allow the head to balance freely on top of the spine, sense the crown of the head lengthening up to the ceiling.

Chest Expansion Plus Rotation

This is more challenging as you have to control rotating to one side while staying centred. Visualise the body's three main weights, head, ribcage and pelvis, balanced on top of each other and swivelling around your central axis. *Suitable for...* All stages.

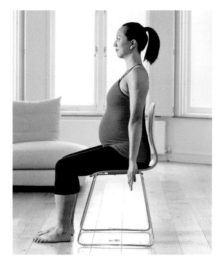

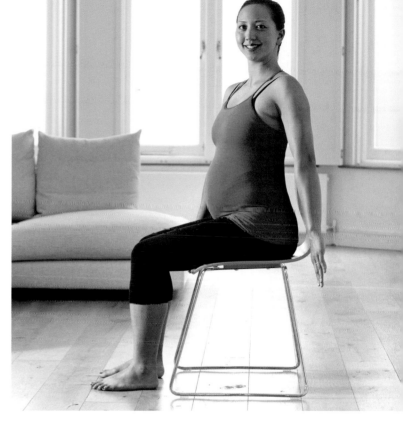

Starting position...

Sit on a chair, Stand Tall, or High Kneel. Hold the weights (if using) lengthening your arms down by the sides of your body with your palms facing backwards, just slightly in front of you.

Zip up to maintain a constant and appropriate connection to your centre throughout.

Action...

1 Breathe in as you press your left arm behind you while simultaneously turning your head, neck and spine to the left. Your right arm may react by swinging forward. Try to turn around your central axis. Keep your pelvis facing forward if possible.

2 Breathe out as you return your trunk, neck, head and arms to the starting position. Repeat to the other side.

Repeat *up to 3 times to each side.*

✳ Watchpoints

– Think of spiralling up up up up, especially as you turn back.

– Do not fix your pelvis, try to keep it steady but if it moves with you, that is fine too.

– Keep both sides of your waist equally long.

– Move slowly and with control.

Chest Extension

As your bump grows, it will become difficult for you to do back extensions lying on your front. Yet it is important that you include some form of back extension in your workout to compensate for any forward bending you have done in your daily activities. *Suitable for...* All stages.

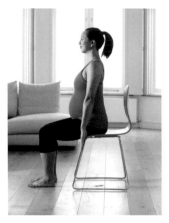

Note Avoid this exercise if you have lumbar-sacral problems. Stop at any time if you feel dizzy.

Starting position...

Sit tall on a sturdy chair, towards the front, feet firmly planted hip-width apart (or wherever they are comfortable). Have your arms lengthened by your sides, gently pressing back into the base of the chair.
Zip up to maintain a constant and appropriate connection to your centre throughout.

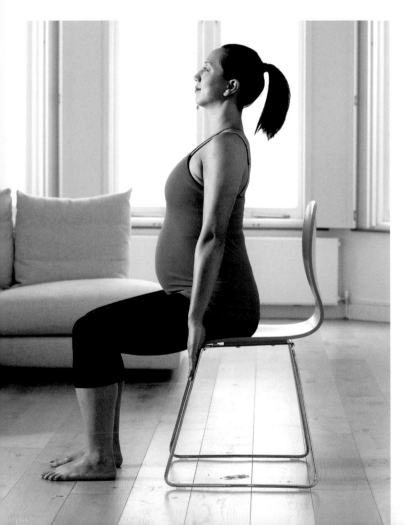

Action...

1 Breathe in to prepare and lengthen up through the spine.
2 Breathe out and gently expand your chest, opening from the base of your throat down through your breastbone. Imagine there is a cord attached to your breastbone, pulling it forward and up, opening the chest towards the ceiling. Your gaze can follow an arc and will stop where the wall meets the ceiling. Do not go back too far, do not tip your head back. Your neck stays long.
3 Breathe in and then, as you breathe out, slowly come to upright again, taking your gaze back down in an arc to where you started.
Repeat *up to 5 times.*

✳ Watchpoints
–   Take care that you extend only your upper back, do not take the extension into your lower back.
–   Your ribs will open but do not allow them to pop out. Think of the rib connection made in Ribcage Closure, page 202.
–   Feet stay planted into the floor.
–   Move slowly and with control.
–   Do not tip the head back too far it should move naturally with the movement of the spine.

Dumb Waiter

A wonderful exercise that helps to encourage release and openness across the front of the chest and shoulders, areas which can become quite tight when you are pregnant due to the heavier weight of the breasts pulling you over into a more rounded posture. *Suitable for...* All stages.

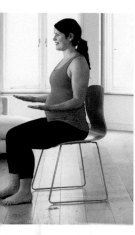

Starting position...

Standing or sitting tall. Bend your elbows and hold your hands out as if holding a tray.

Zip up to maintain a constant and appropriate connection to your centre throughout.

Action...

1   Breathe in and keeping your elbows directly underneath your shoulders, turn your arms outwards from the shoulder joint, reaching your forearms wide.

2   Breathe out as you return the arms back to the Starting position; your forearms once again parallel.

Repeat *up to 10 times.*

Variation

For a change try this version which will help your co-ordination and balance. Follow the directions as above, but this time, only open one arm to the side while simultaneously turning your head the other way. Lengthen up as you turn the head, keep your gaze on one level.

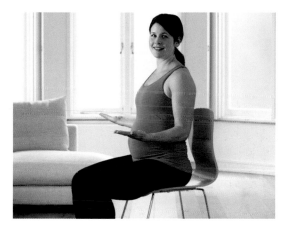

> ## * Watchpoints
>
> – Lengthen up through the crown of your head.
>
> – Ensure that the movement comes from the shoulder joint alone, do not squeeze your shoulder-blades together, and instead focus on them remaining wide across the back of your ribcage.
>
> – Keep your fingers and hands lengthened and ensure that they remain aligned with your forearm.

Seated Scapular Squeeze

Another chest opener, but this time in a seated position. This position may be used during the first stage of labour as it also encourages the baby to descend and helps to open the pelvis. *Suitable for...* All stages. **Equipment** A sturdy chair without arms and with a seat that isn't too wide.

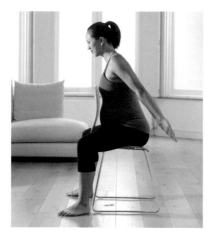

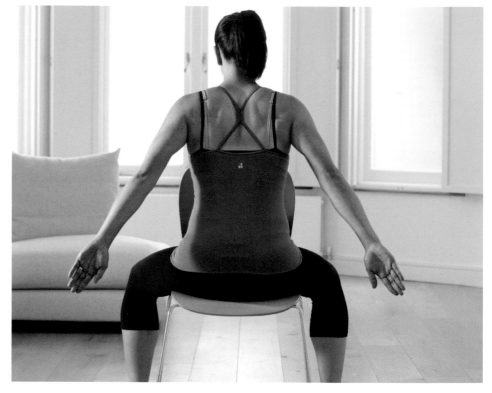

Starting position...

Either sit astride the chair the wrong way round or if the seat is too wide or your bump too big, sit the right way round. Either way you should feel very comfortable in this position. Your legs are turned out from your hips (to allow bump room) but both feet should be firmly planted on the ground.

Zip up to maintain a constant and appropriate connection to your centre throughout.

Action...

1 Hinge forward from the hips, moving your body as one unit from the hip joints themselves. Think long and strong, arms are lengthened down out behind you, palms facing backwards.

2 Breathe in and take your arms wide to the sides opening out the collar-bones.

✳ Watchpoints

– Keep lengthening, lengthening, lengthening the spine. Create space for your baby.

– Take care not to tip the head back. The neck stays long and in line with the spine. In fact as the arms squeeze together you should feel your neck lengthen into freedom like a turtle emerging from its shell.

– You should feel the work between the shoulder-blades and at the back of the arms.

– Try not to twist the wrists or hands; keep them in line.

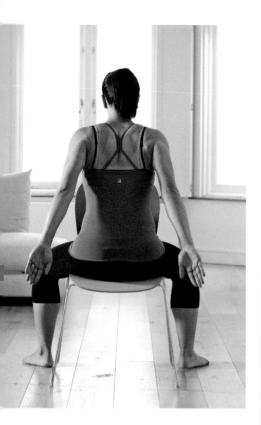

Wrist Circles

A simple but effective exercise for mobilising the wrist joints. It is a good way to release tension around the forearm. *Suitable for...* All stages.

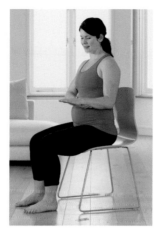

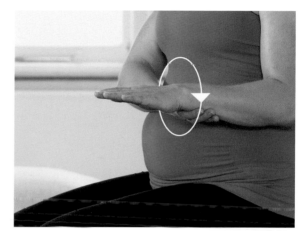

3 Breathe out and squeeze the shoulder-blades together bringing the arms towards each other but keeping them straight.

4 Breathe in and take the lengthened arms back wide again.

Repeat *up to 6 times before hinging back to upright.*

Starting position...

Sit tall on a chair or mat. Bend one arm at the elbow, the hand will be palm down and support the elbow with your other hand. Keep your upper body open.

Action...

1 Keeping your shoulders relaxed and your upper arms still, begin to circle your wrist inwards and around, completing a full, even circle. Keep fingers lengthened and free from tension.

2 Repeat the wrist circle five times and then reverse the direction and circle the wrist five times outwards.

Repeat *with the other hand.*

✳ Watchpoints

– Breathe naturally throughout and allow your core muscles to relax.

– Ensure that the movement comes from the wrist joint and does not involve the fingers.

– Try to keep your upper arm still, your forearm will rotate a little.

– Remain lengthened in your neck, open in the chest and relaxed in your shoulders. If you do feel any tension in your shoulders then try lowering your arm slightly.

– Attempt to create full and even circles.

Arm Openings

More opening for the chest... This is a truly fabulous feel-good exercise which mobilises the head, neck and torso through a balanced rotational movement. This movement is coupled with a smooth and flowing arm movement that promotes openness and control around the shoulders. *Suitable for...* All stages.

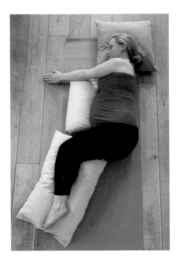 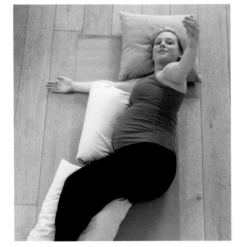 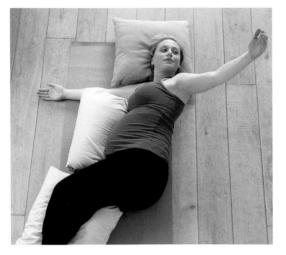

Starting position...

Lie on your right side. Place a pillow underneath the head to align it with your neck and spine. Bend both knees in front of you so that your hips and knees are bent at a right angle. Place another pillow between the knees and ankles and another under your bump or waist. Lengthen both arms out in front of your body at shoulder height.

Zip up to maintain a constant and appropriate connection to your centre throughout.

Action...

1 Breathe in as you raise the top arm, keeping it straight and lifting it above the shoulder joint towards the ceiling, simultaneously roll your head and neck to face the ceiling.

2 Breathe out as you continue to rotate your head, neck and upper spine to the left, carry your left arm with your spine and open it further towards the mat. Your knees and pelvis remain still.

3 Breathe in as you rotate your spine back to the right, initiating the movement from your centre. Simultaneously reach your left arm once again above the shoulder joint and towards the ceiling.

4 Breathe out as you rotate and return your spine and arm back to the Starting position.

Repeat *up to 8 times, and then repeat on the other side.*

✳ Watchpoints

- Ensure correct alignment in your side-lying starting position: shoulder above shoulder, hip above hip, knee above knee and foot above foot.
- Ensure that your pelvis remains stable throughout.
- As you rotate, continue to lengthen the spine; avoid arching in your back or shortening in your waist.
- Do not allow your arms to move beyond the rotation of the spine.
- Keep lengthening through the crown of the head both as you open and close the arms.
- Fully lengthen your arms, but avoid locking your elbows.

Oyster

This opens the hips, and helps strengthen your deep gluteals, stabilising your pelvis. A good one to firm up your buttocks! *Suitable for...* All stages. Take medical advice if you have pelvic girdle pain (see page 193). Postnatal, if you have had a caesarean section, open the knee carefully and not so far that it pulls on the scar.

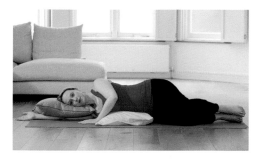

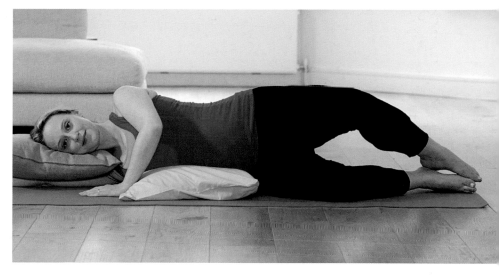

Starting position...

Side-lying on your right, in a straight line, stacking your shoulders, hips and ankles. Pelvis and spine in neutral. Lengthen your right arm underneath and in line with your spine, you will probably need a flat cushion or folded towel under your head. Place your left hand on the mat in front of you and bend your elbow to help lightly support your position. Bend both knees so that your heels are aligned with the back of your pelvis.

If you are in the later stages of pregnancy, you may wish to place one pillow under your bump or waist and another between your knees.

Zip up to maintain a constant and appropriate connection to your centre throughout.

Action...

1   Breathe in, preparing your body to move.

2   Breathe out as you open your top knee keeping your feet connected together. This 'turn out' movement will come from your hip joint. Keep your pelvis still and stable.

3   Breathe in and with control return your leg to the Starting position.

Repeat *up to 10 times and then repeat on the other side.*

✳ Watchpoints

–   To help reach the right muscles, try gently squeezing your heels together. Make sure that both heels squeeze evenly.

–   Open your top leg only as far as you can without disturbing the position of your pelvis.

–   Keep lengthening both sides of the waist throughout.

–   The top arm is positioned to help support you, but avoid placing too much weight onto it.

–   Keep your chest open, and your focus directly ahead of you.

Walking on the Spot

A wonderful exercise for working the feet, ankles and calves, while also waking up your circulation in the legs, which helps prevent swelling. If you ever find yourself stuck standing in a queue or on a bus or train and you start to feel dizzy but there's nowhere to sit down, try this as it gets the deep calf pump working and your blood flowing.

The key to doing this exercise well is to keep good body alignment throughout. You have three main body weights, your head, your ribcage and your pelvis. Try to keep them balanced centrally on top of each other. When you bend your knees in this exercise the knees should bend directly over the second toes. You may have to check this occasionally during the exercise. *Suitable for...* All stages.

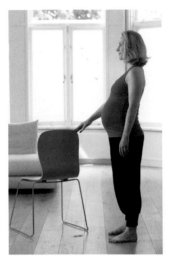 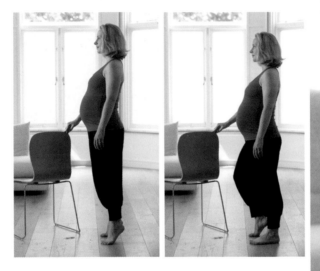

Starting position...

Stand tall. You may need to hold onto a wall or the back of a high chair. Your feet are almost together.
Zip up to maintain a constant and appropriate connection to your centre throughout.

Action...

Breathing normally, rise up onto the balls of both feet, then lower one heel down, stay on the ball of the other foot, the knee bends slightly then change legs transferring your weight, but not wiggling your hips. Keep lengthening up, up, up and keep the waist long.
Continue *'walking' on the spot for a couple of minutes.*

✳ **Watchpoints**

– Think up, up, up take care not to sink down onto one side.

– Try to keep your pelvis level, waist equally long on both sides. No wiggling.

– Use your core muscles to hold up your bump.

– Check every so often that your knees are bending straight over your second toes.

– Keep the action smooth and flowing.

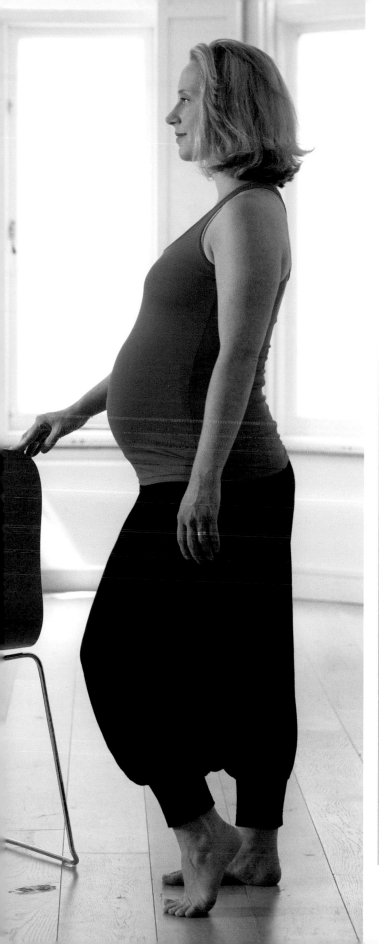

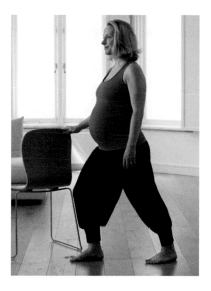

Calf Stretch

There is a possibility that you will be suffering from leg cramps, particularly at night. This exercise may help. *Suitable for...* All stages.

Starting position and Action...

1 Stand alongside a wall or sturdy chair.

2 Place hand on the chair or wall for support.

3 Bend one knee, then take a step back with the other foot. Stay facing forwards. This back leg should be straight but not locked at the knee. The toes should be pointing forward and the heel down creating a stretch in the calf muscles. Keep the weight spread evenly through the feet between the big toe, small toe and heel.

4 Hold this stretch for about 20 seconds before releasing the stretch and stepping back.

Repeat *with the other leg.*

✳ Watchpoints
- Keep lengthening upwards.
- Your front foot should face forward, the knee bent in line with the ankle.

Seated Zig Zags

Another great exercise for increasing mobility in the hips joints while trying to maintain a stable relationship between the hip, knee and ankle joints. It also challenges the stability of your spine as the legs move independently from the hips. You will be making a zig-zag pattern with your feet. *Suitable for...* All stages.

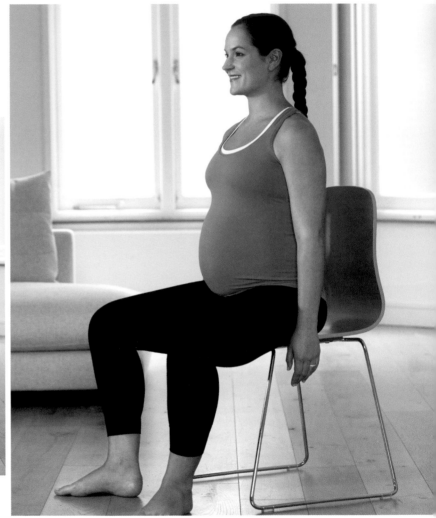

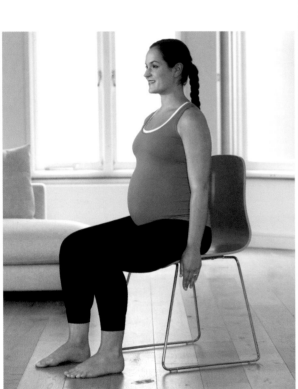

Starting position...

Sit upright on a sturdy chair. You will need to be near the front of the seat, have your arms lengthened alongside you. Have your legs slightly wider than hip-width.

Zip up to maintain a constant and appropriate connection to your centre throughout.

Action...

1 Breathe in and lengthen your spine.

2 Breathe out and turn your thigh bones outwards from the hips. Your knees and feet will also turn out.

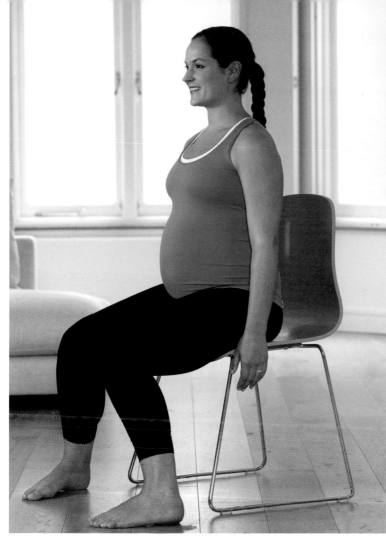

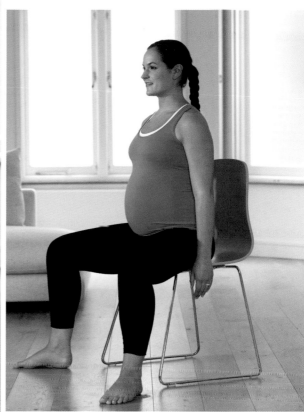

4 Breathe out and turn the thighs bones out.

5 Keep turning in and out as far as comfortable and then start turning back in…and out…until you return to the Starting position.

Repeat *up to 5 times.*

3 Breathe in and now turn your thigh bones in from the hips. Once again the knees and feet react by turning in also.

✻ Watchpoints

– Keep the weight even on both sitting bones throughout.

– Keep your pelvis and spine stable; focus on the independent movement of the thigh bones in the hip sockets.

– Control the movement of your legs and don't just allow them to 'drop' in and out.

– It is easy to let your feet or your knees turn out, or in, further than your hips can turn out, but it is essential that this be avoided.

– Keep your chest and the front of your shoulders open and avoid any tension in your neck area.

Side-lying Circles

This exercise follows on from Oyster; once again we are looking to mobilise the hips while strengthening the gluteals. It will also challenge your core as you are aiming to keep your trunk steady. *Suitable for...* All stages. Take advice if you have pelvic girdle pain (page 193).

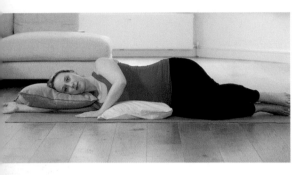

Starting position...

Lie on your right side in a straight line, stacking your shoulders and hips but with your legs bent and forward as if you are sitting on a chair. If in the later stages of pregnancy, place a pillow under your bump or waist and another between your legs (optional). Have your head resting on your outstretched lower arm in line with your body. You can place a flat pillow under your head if you wish as long as the neck stays in line with the spine.

Zip up to maintain a constant and appropriate connection to your centre throughout.

Action...

1 Lift your left leg so that it is level with the top of your pelvis and bring it back in line with your hip. Straighten your leg, keeping it parallel. Softly point your foot.

2 Breathe at your normal pace as you lengthen and circle the leg around in an anti-clockwise direction.

3 Repeat up to five circles in the same direction (one breath for each circle) and then change to circle the leg clockwise.

Repeat *twice and then turn over to repeat on the other side. When you are finished, bend your leg and bring it forward to rest back in the Starting position with control. Do not just drop the leg down.*

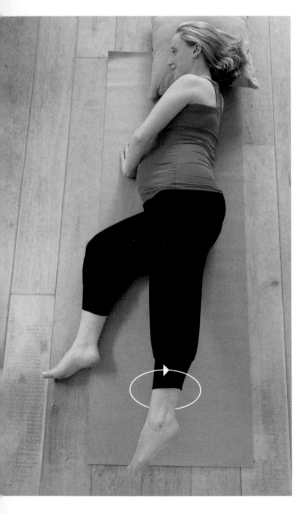

> ## ✳ Watchpoints
>
> – The circle is small, about the size of a grapefruit. Keep the circle even, i.e. as far as you carry the leg forward, you must carry it the same distance behind you. Do not dip the leg lower than hip height.
>
> – Maintain the parallel position of your leg throughout the circle.
>
> – Stay active in your middle, do not slump there, both sides of your waist lifted and lengthened.
>
> – Keep your chest open and your focus directly ahead of you.
>
> – Ensure that your pelvis remains stable throughout. The action must come from your hip joint, as your leg moves in isolation to the rest your body.
>
> – Keep the underneath leg active – this will help your balance.

The Flower

An important pelvic floor exercise to help you learn how to release this area. *Suitable for...* All stages (Later Pregnancy use a Seated or even your chosen birthing position).

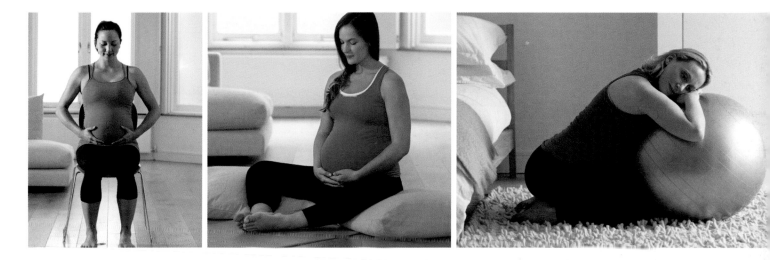

Starting position...

Seated on a mat or chair or by the wall Four-point Kneeling position, or you can even try this in a birthing position. Think of your favourite flower!

Action...

1   Breathe in and prepare your body.

2   Breathe out as you gather together and gradually draw up the muscles of your pelvic floor inside you; imagining a flower closing tightly like a bud.

3   Breathe in and gently hold the flower closed.

4   Breathe out as you slowly allow the flower to completely open, blowing air out gently through your mouth as you do so.

5   Breathe in and ever so slightly close the flower, to return the pelvic floor to its normal tone.

Repeat *up to 6 times.*

NB You can vary the breathing pattern if you wish if it helps you release better on the in-breath.

✱ Watchpoints

–   Keep your jaw and mouth soft. Have your lips gently open.

–   If you wish, you may practise releasing your pelvic floor as you breathe out and blow out onto the back of your hand.

–   Ensure that your pelvis remains still throughout, the subtle opening of the flower is purely internal; make sure that you keep your buttock muscles relaxed.

–   Continue to breathe fully throughout – it is very important not to hold your breath.

–   Keep your chest and the front of your shoulders open and avoid any tension in your neck area.

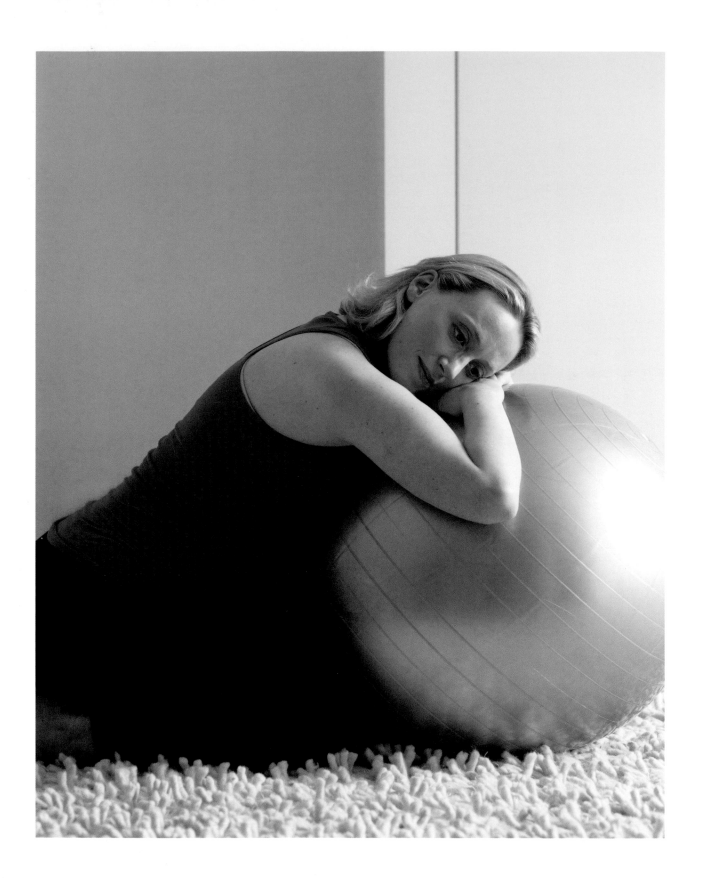

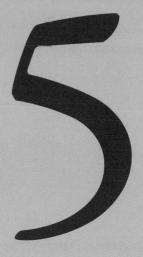

Preparing for Labour and the Birth

Preparing for Labour and the Birth

After months of waiting, the big day approaches and, naturally, you want to be as ready as you can be. This does not just mean having your bag packed or plastic sheets on the bed! It means that your mind and your body should be prepared. Stamina is one of our guiding principles and, if you have been exercising regularly over the last few months, you will have helped improve yours in readiness for the task ahead. It helps to know what to expect and to have worked out a game plan. This chapter will highlight ways in which your Pilates practice can help supplement any antenatal training your chosen clinic may provide.

We will briefly cover what happens in the three stages of labour. In the reference section at the back of the book you will find listed some books which can give you more comprehensive information. Our focus is on how to use your Pilates skills to make your labour and delivery as easy and comfortable as possible.

Labour

When it comes to advice on how to manage your labour, you will find that there are many different schools of thought. Each mother should consult her medical practitioner/midwife/doula as to which type of birthing method will best suit their particular pregnancy. You may decide on a home or hospital birth. You may decide to attend classes to learn a particular birthing plan such as the Lamaze Method, Bradley Method, Read Method, Active Birth Method, Mongan Method (Hypnobirthing), Autogenic or Odent Method, to name but a few!

Whatever you choose, bear in mind that no two pregnancies or births are the same so you need to be prepared for all eventualities. Do not be disappointed if things do not go according to plan. Even the best prepared mothers can have births which do not stick to the script!

The more in tune you are with your body, the more you will understand what is happening. The fitter you are and the more stamina you have, the better you will be able to manage the birth process. Labour is, as the word suggests, hard work but it is also what our bodies have been designed to do!

If you can be flexible and adapt according to what is happening, then you stay in control. Practice makes all the difference. Research confirms this showing, for example, that if you practise your pelvic floor exercises throughout your pregnancy you may have a shorter second stage of labour.

Let's look first at what will be happening during labour.
Labour is normally described as having three phases:
1 The dilation of the cervix. At the end of this first stage is the transitional period.
2 The delivery, the expulsion of the baby – the birth.
3 The expulsion of the placenta and membranes.

First Stage of Labour Over the last weeks of pregnancy you will probably have felt some practice or Braxton Hicks contractions. If this is your first pregnancy at some time during the last six weeks your baby's head may have engaged down into the pelvic inlet. It does not always happen. You are considered to be in the first stage of labour when your cervix is 3cm dilated and you are having regular strong contractions.

There are many early signs of labour, including the loss of the mucous plug, a pink thick discharge, leaking pale amniotic fluid. But some mothers wait for a show and never have one and sometimes the mucous plug comes out stuck on the top of the baby's head! So perhaps the best indicators are the contractions themselves, which will become stronger and more frequent. The contractions come in waves as the uterus contracts, the cervix thins and draws up, slowly opening.

If you think you are going into labour, or when your contractions are 5–7 minutes apart, it is worth giving your midwife/hospital/doula some advance warning. They can then tell you at what point you should go to hospital or attend you at home.

Call your midwife/doctor immediately if you experience any of the following:

∗ Discharge of bright red blood

∗ Strong contractions when your due date is a long way off

∗ Your waters break but you have no contractions

∗ If your waters break and are green or brown in colour

∗ You notice something in your vagina. It may be the umbilical cord, so call an ambulance immediately.

How long this first stage will last is not predictable. Some women go from 0–60 in a matter of an hour! If this is your first baby, it may last 8–16 hours. For a second or subsequent baby this stage is usually shorter.

By the end of this first stage, your cervix needs to be open 10cm to allow the baby to be delivered – just a bit smaller in circumference than a DVD or CD.

Now, 8–16 hours is a long time to be coping with regular, strong contractions. You need to discuss with your midwife how you are going to manage this stage. Ideally, you will be able to move around. It is unlikely that you will want to stay in one position. First and second stages of labour have been shown to be shorter if the mother remains upright, with mothers reporting greater comfort, more control and less pain.

There are many advantages to staying upright during labour. Your uterus tilts forward as it contracts, so if you can stay in an upright position, gravity can assist it. Thankfully gone are the days when you had to lie still on your back and the uterus had to fight gravity while the baby travelled uphill! It stands to reason that any muscle working against gravity will fatigue more quickly.

The dilation of the cervix

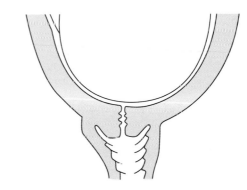

No dilation

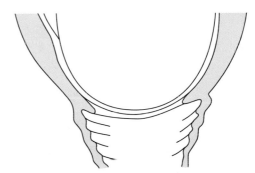

Dilation nearly complete

Furthermore, we have already seen how leaning forward helps to open up the pelvis, allowing the baby an easier route to descend through the pelvic canal, so squatting positions and supported squats are very useful. If your baby is still breech (see below), just check with your midwife before squatting.

The ligamentous laxity we have been referring to throughout the book was for a reason. It allows the pelvic joints to expand and move according to the shape of the baby's head as it descends. This process is much easier if the mother is in an upright position as the joints are not compressed.

A squatting position allows the sacrum to move freely. The sacrococcygeal joint between the sacrum and coccyx (your tailbone) can swivel backwards widening the outlet as the baby emerges, but this is not so easy if the mother is sitting on her coccyx. The perineum can also expand more evenly and pull back (like a turtle neck) over the baby's head as it emerges, helping to reduce the need for an episiotomy or the risk of tearing.

Studies have shown that a mother's contractions are more regular and frequent when she stays upright. The cervix is believed to dilate more efficiently as it responds to the extra pressure of the baby's head (or presenting part) and gravity on the cervix. Circulation within the placenta is improved in an upright position, allowing better oxygen flow to the baby. Incidence of foetal distress is lower and the baby's condition once born is reported as better.

You can relax in an upright position and still be very comfortable. A good chair or the large inflatable ball are very useful!

Exercises such as Pilates Squats, Hip Hinge, Seated Scapular Squeeze and Wall Slides are all excellent preparation for remaining upright in labour. You will want to feel comfortable in your squat position, which requires some 'thigh power' and flexibility around the hips.

If your knees are healthy, then you might like to practise deeper squats with a partner. These deeper squat positions will stretch your perineum in readiness for when your baby's head emerges.

Avoid practising deep squats if you have any knee or ankle problems, varicose veins or piles.

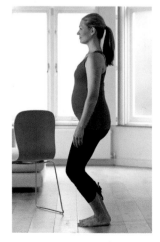 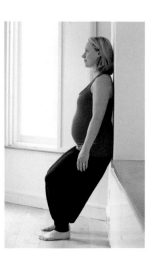 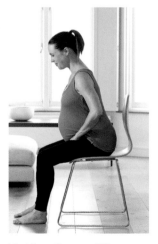 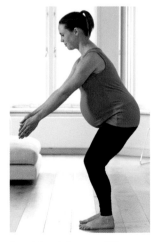

Tennis Ball Rising *See page 127*   Wall Slides *See page 210*   Hip Hinge *See page 152*   Squat Squat *See page 153*

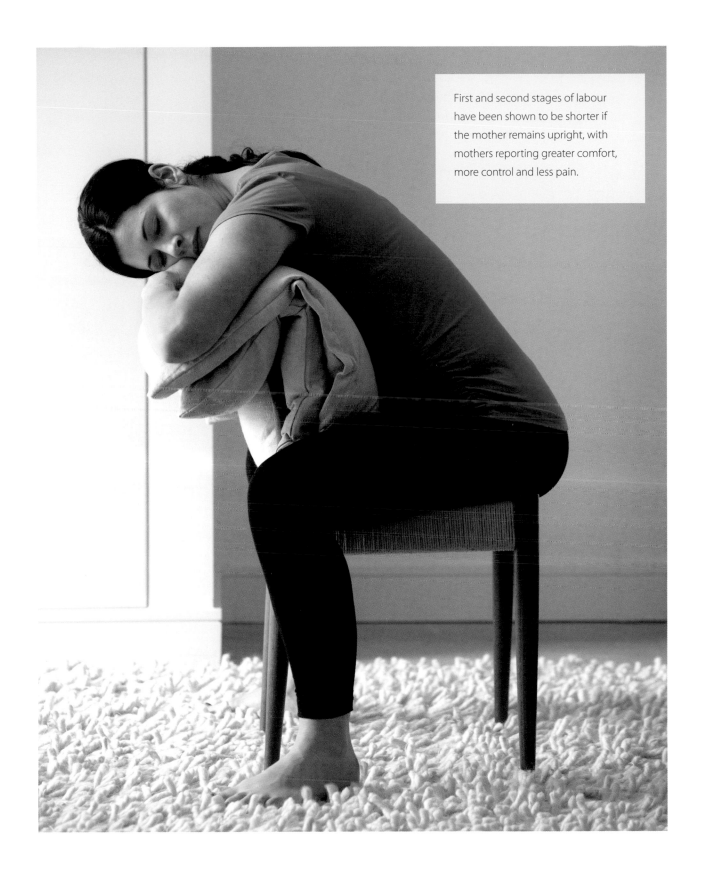

First and second stages of labour have been shown to be shorter if the mother remains upright, with mothers reporting greater comfort, more control and less pain.

Partner Squatting

The going down is the easy bit, it's the coming back up that proves the challenge! *Suitable for...* Early and Later Pregnancy. Take advice if your baby is breech presentation from 35 weeks on. Squatting places a lot of strain on the knees. Caution with knee problems, varicose veins and piles.

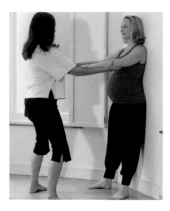

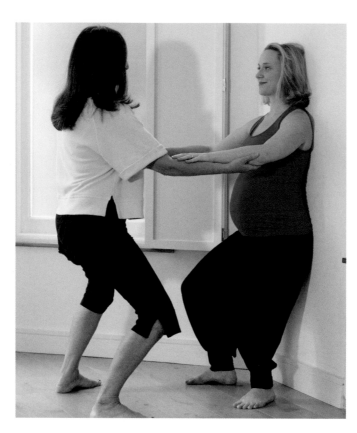

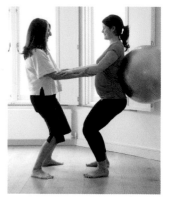

Starting position...
Stand in the Wall Slide Position, with your feet wider apart than normal and turned out from the hips. Your partner mirrors your position facing you. Hold each other's forearms firmly. Partner follows the directions too!
Zip up to maintain a constant and appropriate connection to your centre throughout.

Variation
Partner squatting with ball
You can also try this exercise in Wall Slide Position with a large Swiss ball behind your back.

Action...
1 Breathe in wide to prepare.
2 Breathe out, slowly lower down into a squat.
3 Breathe in then out and with your partner still holding on slowly slide back up the wall.
Repeat *up to 8 times.*

Free-standing Partner Squats

These squats have the advantage of allowing you to hip hinge forward as you squat. *Suitable for...* Early and Later Pregnancy. Take advice if your baby is breech presentation from 35 weeks on. Caution with knee problems and varicose veins or piles.

Action...

1 Breathe in wide to prepare.

2 Breathe out and slowly lower down into a squat. Hinge forward if you wish.

3 Breathe in, then out and press the floor away with both feet as you come back up.

Repeat *up to 8 times.*

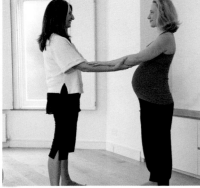

Starting position...

Stand facing each other. Legs apart, slightly turned out from the hips. Your partner holds your forearms firmly.

Zip up to maintain a constant and appropriate connection to your centre throughout.

✳ Watchpoints

– Direct your knees over the centre of your feet.

– Lengthen from your tailbone to the top of your head.

– Do not to allow your knees or ankles to buckle in or out.

– As you straighten up, press the floor away evenly through the soles of both feet.

– Keep the heels in contact with the floor if you can.

– Keep the waist long.

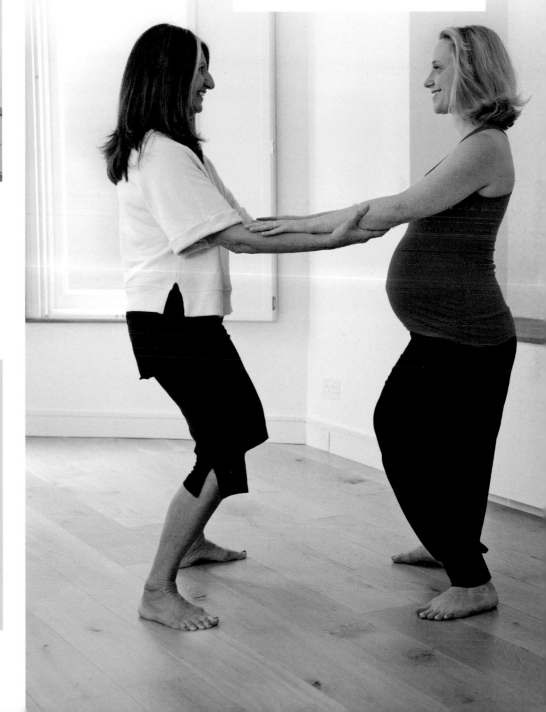

Relaxation During Labour

As we have mentioned, this first stage can last up to 16 hours and you want to save some energy for the pushing bit! The last thing you want is to go into your second stage exhausted. So your focus will be on staying as relaxed as possible so that the uterus can get on with its job unhindered. This means keeping an eye on unwanted tension creeping between contractions and during contractions.

Learning how to release tension is a skill which can be mastered. Of course it is one thing releasing tension during a Pilates session, quite another trying to stay relaxed during strong contractions. It will be challenging.

Think of useful Pilates cues...

✳ Focus on the ebb and flow of your breathing.

✳ Allow your collar bones to widen.

✳ Allow your shoulders to melt.

✳ Allow your joints to open.

With each contraction, try to visualise your cervix softening and opening. Think of a flower opening in the same way as you did for The Flower exercise on page 167 (only this time it will not be closing).

There is no reason why you cannot do a few gentle release exercises such as Shoulder Drops, Neck Rolls, as long as you adapt a safe position. When trying to find a comfortable position to relax you may need to experiment. We know that lying flat on your back is not an option due to supine hypotensive syndrome. Some centres have specially designed cushions that allow you to rest on your front. Some centres have birthing balls which are the large balls that we use in Pilates classes. You may be allowed to bring your own ball into the labour room.

You could try kneeling forward over a pile of cushions. Alternatively you could use a propped up seated position or side-lying (see pictures below). Many beds in labour wards or birthing centres have a setting which brings the mother into an upright seated squat.

For relaxation during this first stage of labour try the Labour Relaxation Position and the Tension Release exercise.

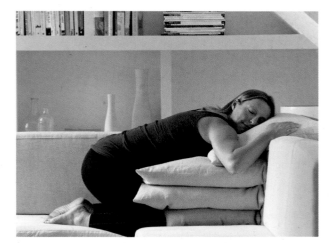

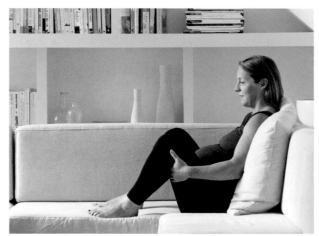

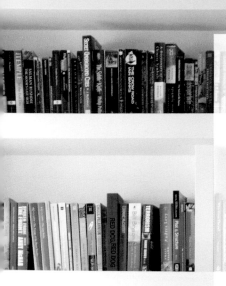
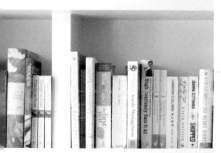

Labour relaxation position

This is a useful rest position during your first stage.

* You need to find a position where you feel properly supported and balanced.
* Stack pillows up either behind you on your bed or against a wall.
* Try a side-lying position and if possible lie on your left side.
* Have your head on a flat pillow, with the chin directed slightly downwards to ensure that your head does not tilt back.
* Your bottom leg is stretched out, but still slightly bent. Your uppermost leg will be bent and resting on two pillows placed lengthwise to support more of the leg; we are trying to keep your pelvis in neutral (hip over hip). The top knee should be in line with the top hip.
* Your underneath arm and shoulder will rest on the bed, the top arm and shoulder will relax forward naturally.
* You should feel really supported and comfortable. Your spine should retain its natural curves.
* If you can relax in this position, you can allow the uterus to contract and get on with the job in hand!

You can simply rest in this position or you can go through a relaxation exercise (or even better you can get your birthing partner to go through the cues for you).
Or try the Tension Release exercise on the next page.

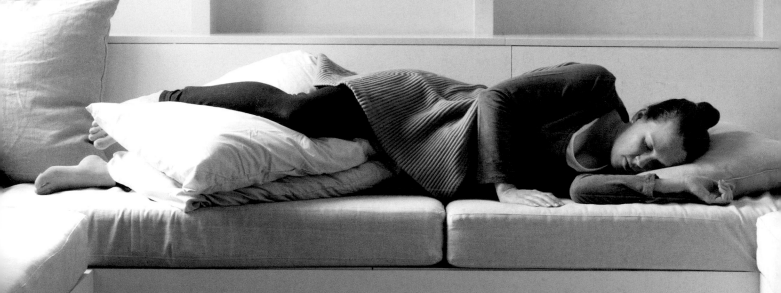

Tension Release Exercise

A systematic relaxation exercise. Try to get someone with a calm, deep gentle voice to record the cues for you.
Suitable for... All stages of pregnancy. Especially helpful in first stage of labour.

Starting position...

Later pregnancy and first stage of labour

Side-lying, or a propped up seated position. Supported Hip Hinged position.

For preparing for pregnancy, early pregnancy and postnatal

You may prefer to lie on your back with a pillow under your head and another under your knees.

✳ Take your awareness down to your feet and soften the soles, uncurling the toes.

✳ Soften your ankles.

✳ Soften your calves.

✳ Release your knees.

✳ Release your thighs.

✳ Allow your hips to open.

✳ Allow the small of your back to open and release.

✳ Feel and enjoy the length of your spine but let it go.

✳ Take your awareness down to your hands, stretch your fingers away from your palms, feel the centre of your palms opening.

✳ Then allow the fingers to curl, the palms to soften.

✳ Allow your elbows to open.

✳ Allow the front of your shoulders to soften.

✳ With each out-breath allow your shoulder blades to widen.

✳ Allow your breastbone to soften.

✳ Allow your neck to release.

✳ Check your jaw, it should be loose and free.

✳ Allow your tongue to widen at its base and rest comfortably at the bottom of your mouth.

✳ Your lips are softly closed.

✳ Dribble if you want to.

✳ Your eyes are softly closed.

✳ Enjoy the soft darkness.

✳ Your forehead is wide and smooth and completely free of lines.

✳ Your face feels soft.

✳ Your body soft and warm.

✳ Allow your body to sink into the pillows supporting you.

✳ Observe your breathing, but do not interrupt its natural rhythm...

If you are in labour...

Relax your abdomen, allow your bump to sag and drift away.
As a contraction builds, let your bump go... allow it to be limp and soft. Let the uterus do the work... you can let go... visualise your cervix opening, your baby descending.

To come out of the relaxation...

Bring your awareness back to your breathing and observe its ebb and flow. Wriggle your fingers... and then your toes. Take your time to move slowly when moving out of your Relaxation.

Baby presentations
and how Pilates may help

During your antenatal visits your doctor/midwife will be checking the position of your baby. This becomes increasingly important as the delivery day approaches. Your baby may choose several different options for which part he or she will present first to the world. Some may make the delivery a little more complicated.

Anterior Presentation Before labour begins, normally a baby will lie with its head engaged in the pelvis in an anterior position. That is, the baby's spine lies in the hammock of the mother's abdominal wall. The baby's limbs are folded in front, facing the mother's spine. Baby's head is tucked well in, ready for a quick and easy exit!

Posterior Presentation Of course some babies haven't read the rule book and decide to face the other way, with their spine against the mother's spine and their limbs folded in towards the mother's abdominal wall. This position may make the delivery more difficult and require instrumental assistance. It can cause a prolonged labour, with contractions felt in the back rather than the front. Most babies rotate naturally into the anterior position during the first stage of labour but sometimes they need an incentive.

Your midwife may ask you to lie on your left side for periods, or stand with one leg abducted to the side on a

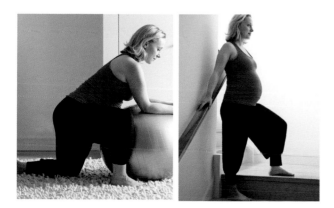

step or kneel (see photos) to help increase the mid-pelvic spaces to encourage rotation.

Or adopt a Four-point Kneeling position. This can be leaning onto a chair or large ball. This position creates more space for the baby to rotate as the uterus hangs in the hammock of the mother's abdomen, and then gravity will encourage the heaviest part of your baby, the spine and the back of the head, to rotate downwards into the desired anterior position.

Breech This is when your baby decides to present bottom or legs first! You can deliver a baby vaginally this way but a breech birth does add extra complications and often a caesarean section is recommended. If you want to deliver your baby vaginally, we want to persuade your baby to come out head first if possible.

You may be advised to use Four-point Kneeling to persuade the baby to turn. Walking for an hour a day helps as the head is the heaviest part of your baby, gravity will help encourage it to move downwards. Just remember that even the most awkwardly positioned babies often leave it to the last minute to turn of their own accord.

While squatting may be used during the second stage to help deliver a baby it may not be helpful earlier. If your baby is breech at 35 weeks, talk to your doctor/midwife. They may advise you to stop squatting as you don't want baby's bottom or legs to engage into the pelvic inlet.

Transverse This is when your baby is lying in a sideways position. You may follow the same advice as for breech babies. Kneeling and rotating your hips may also help. But it is unlikely that the baby will turn of its own accord. An obstetrician may try to turn the baby in utero but in most cases they will recommend a caesarian section.

Your doctor/midwife will monitor the baby's position during the later stages of your pregnancy and labour.

Four-point Kneeling Exercises

Four-point Kneeling is an incredibly useful position throughout your pregnancy but particularly towards the end and during labour as it encourages the baby to turn. This position can be tough on your wrists but as we have been practising it throughout the whole programme, your wrists should be strong enough to support you for as long as necessary. You can always take a break, sit back and stretch your wrists if needs be (see opposite).

Note though that as your baby grows you will have to use your core muscles to keep the spine in good alignment. You cannot just rest in this position, you need to be active!

Pelvic Clocks in Four-point Kneeling is ideal during labour (see page 92).

In the following two exercises, it helps to visualise your tailbone as a dog's tail. In Pelvic Rocking, you will be tucking your tail under, like a greyhound who is sulking. In Tail Swish, well, the name says it all, you are happy and are going to wag your tail!

Pelvic Rocking

Suitable for... All stages of pregnancy, First stage of labour, Postnatal, but caution in the first few weeks following delivery.

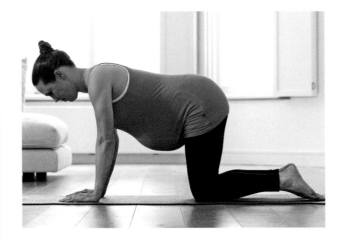

Starting position...
Four-point Kneeling. Position your hands directly underneath your shoulders and your knees directly beneath your hips.
Zip up to maintain a constant and appropriate connection to your centre throughout.

Action...

1 Breathe in, preparing your body to move, and lengthen your spine.

2 Breathe out as you tilt your pelvis, tucking your tailbone under, your pubic bone moves forward, your lower back will slightly round.

3 Breathe in and slowly unravel your spine, sending your tailbone back and away until your pelvis is back level and in neutral.

Repeat *this gentle rocking action 10 times, then settle in back in neutral as shown in Starting position.*

Wrist stretches

This position can be tough on your wrists but as we have been practising it throughout the whole programme, your wrists should be strong enough to support you for as long as necessary. You can always take a break, sit back and stretch your wrists if need be.

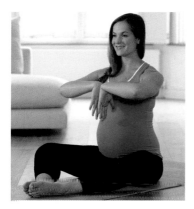

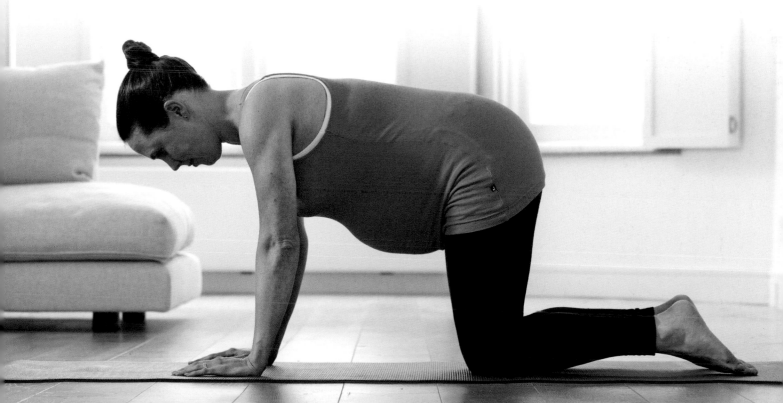

Tail Swish

As with Pelvic Rocking this may be a useful way to encourage your baby to rotate into the desired anterior presentation. *Suitable for...* All stages of pregnancy. Especially useful in the first stage of labour. Postnatal caution in the first few weeks.

Starting position...

Four-point Kneeling. Position your hands directly underneath your shoulders and your knees directly beneath your hips.

Zip up to maintain a constant and appropriate connection to your centre throughout.

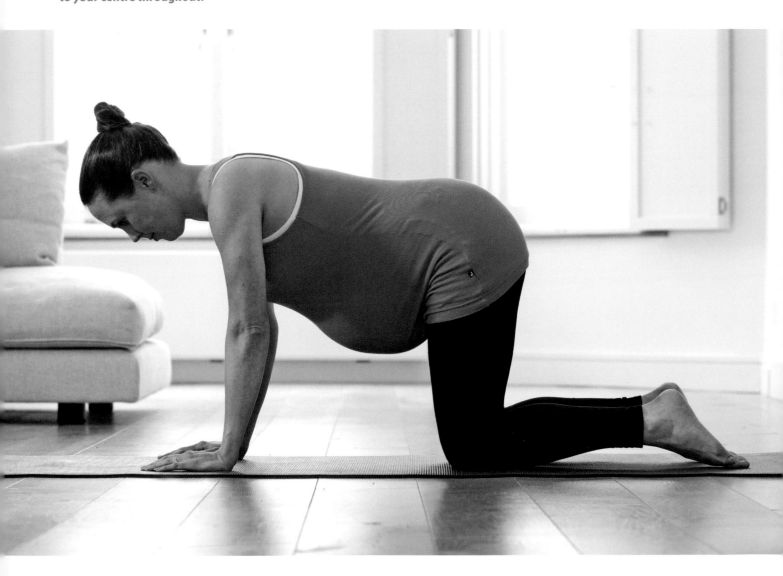

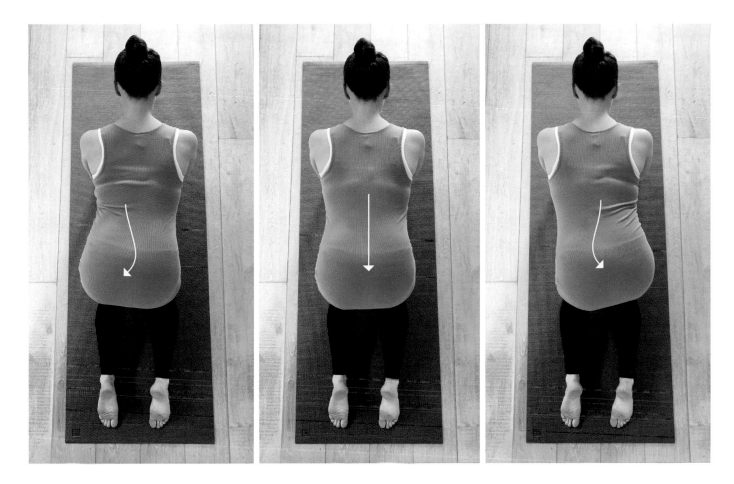

Action...

1 Breathe in to prepare the body, lengthening the spine.

2 Breathe out and wag your tail to your left, drawing the left side of your pelvis towards your left shoulder. Try to keep your pelvis horizontally level with the floor.

3 Breathe in and move your tail back to the centre, returning both sides of your waist to equal length.

4 Breathe out and wag your tail to the right as above.

5 Breathe in and return to the centre.

Repeat *up to 5 times each way.*

* **Watchpoints**

— Inevitably, one side of your waist will shorten as the other lengthens, but try to create length and space on both sides.

— Keep your core connection to avoid your pelvis and spine collapsing down towards the mat.

— Although the movements should be controlled, they should also feel free and released.

— Fully lengthen your arms but avoid locking your elbows.

— Although the focus is on the lower body, remember to keep your chest and the front of your shoulders open and avoid any tension in your neck area.

Transition

Towards the end of this first stage of labour, when you are roughly 8–10cm dilated, you are said to be in transition. The midwife can establish this by examining you internally but usually the best give-away is your mood change. Be prepared for this to be quite dramatic. Your contractions are coming hard and fast, you have very little time to rest between, your whole focus is now on getting this baby born as soon as possible, nothing else matters. You may experience feelings of self-doubt and confusion, hot and cold flushes are common, as is burping, you may shake and tremble or feel nauseous. (Of course you may experience none of these.)

While it may seem as though this will never end, you are very nearly there. The support and encouragement of your birthing partner (if you have one) is crucial here. Even if your birthing partner's efforts are not appreciated at the time (I can remember swearing at my poor husband that he couldn't possibly help as he had no idea what it felt like!) they will be later.

It is important to try to relax all the non-working parts of your body, that is, everywhere except your uterus! Allow the uterus to do its work. If you have learnt a particular birthing method's breathing pattern to help with your contractions, stick with it. If not, then focus on breathing with a quiet and steady rhythm.

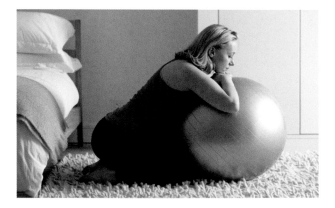

Second stage of labour

It's time to get to work! At last, your cervix is open and you have been given the all-clear to push with your contractions. This second stage can take anything from half an hour to three hours.

While at the end of the first stage your contractions were coming every two minutes, leaving you little rest, your pushing contractions are slightly further apart, leaving you a rest period in between. Make the most of this rest time so you can put all your effort into pushing. Mothers experience different degrees of the urge to push. Some feel it strongly, others less so. The main action of the uterus now is the top moving down on the baby to push them out. The idea is that as the uterus pushes, you increase the force by pushing too, to help the baby move down the birth canal. You normally get 3–5 strong urges to push with each contraction. Make each one count.

Your perineum will stretch during the delivery as your baby's head emerges. Luckily all the squatting will have helped make this area flexible. Your pelvic floor needs to be released and open as your baby is born. We have prepared you for this with pelvic floor releases. Be prepared for the breathing patterns for these exercises and for the delivery to be different.

Whichever position you choose to push in, your legs are going to need to be comfortably apart. We have worked throughout the programme to gently lengthen your inner thighs evenly.

As before, you will want to be in the best possible position to assist your baby's descent. There are lots of options. Upright is best as gravity will assist you. Try different positions before the birth to see which one is comfortable for you as each upright position has its own advantages. Your partner, midwife or doula can help support you in whichever position you chose. You may be limited by what is available in your birthing room or at home or by what is happening to your baby. You may of course change position. If at home you can turn a dining chair to face you as shown opposite, using pillows to support the bump. Or turn the chair upside down and catch hold of the two back feet of the chair. Ideally you would be in a full squat, as the diameter of your pelvic outlet increases by about 1.5cm when your legs are flexed.

If you can remember, gently lengthen the back of your neck and tuck your chin in as you push (the Cervical Nod, page 55). It will help you avoid neck strain.

Breathing during the second stage With your Pilates training, you should now be well connected with your breathing. There are many approaches to how the breath can be used to help push your baby out. If you have been attending birthing classes, follow whichever breathing pattern you have learnt. If, on the other hand, you haven't practised a set pattern, simply trust your natural instincts. Your midwife or doula will cue your breathing if needed.

If you are in an upright squatting or kneeling position, breathing is usually spontaneous. Focus on the out-breath as the contractions start to help you stay relaxed, don't fight the contraction. Think of the Flower opening and releasing. Focusing on your out-breath, breathe the baby down, down, down. Make as much noise as you wish.

Sometimes you may be asked to hold your breath, but normally this is not recommended as it lessens your (and thus your baby's) supply of oxygen. You may be asked to pant as the baby's head crowns, to help the head be delivered more slowly help to prevent a perineal tear.

The most important thing to avoid is hyperventilating (over-breathing) as it may interfere with the uterus's ability to contract. Not only can hyperventilating affect the mother, causing dizziness, blurred vision or tingling or numbness in your fingers and toes it may also reduce the baby's oxygen levels.

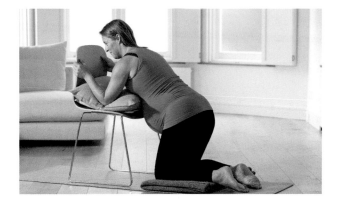

Third stage
Congratulations, you've done it!

Hopefully, you will be able to hold your baby straight away; skin to skin helps you to bond. While you take these few precious first moments getting to know your baby, your uterus will continue to contract. You may not even notice this as the joy of having given birth takes over. Your partner can also experience skin to skin contact with their new child.

The contractions are separating the placenta from the wall of the uterus. Gravity can continue to assist the mother even when her baby is born by helping her placenta and fluids to drain away if she remains upright.

As your baby nurses at your breast, hormones are released which make the uterus contract. Your baby will be taking their first breaths independently with their own lungs. The placenta and umbilical cord continue to pulsate until your baby is breathing normally. This third stage is very important and should not be rushed. It may take an hour for the uterus to expel the placenta. It used to be the practice to pull on the cord to deliver the placenta but normally now the process is allowed to proceed naturally. Some couples like to cut the cord themselves.

If your perineum has torn; or if your midwife gave you an episiotomy, you may need stitching to repair the damage. You will be offered a local anaesthetic to numb the area.

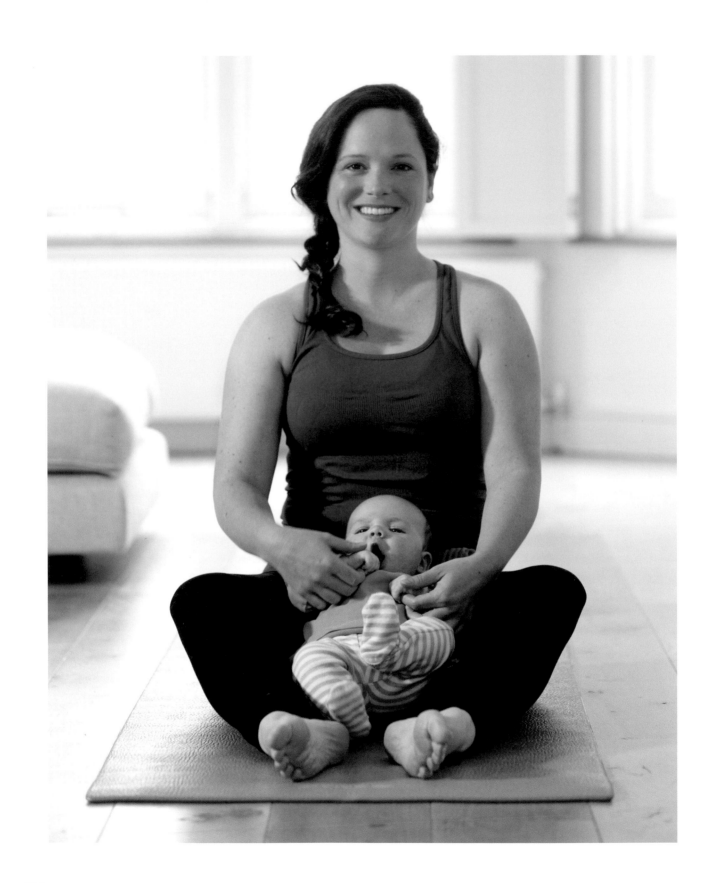

After the Birth

After the Birth

Congratulations! You are a mother!

These first few days and weeks after giving birth are precious. It is a time for you and your family to get to know your newborn baby.

The new life that you have carried within you for nine months is now outside of you, but still totally dependent on you for all its needs. This is a huge responsibility on parents and can be quite a strain. You may also be overwhelmed by visitors as friends, family and neighbours drop by. It's very easy for the baby get all the attention and your needs to be forgotten.

Yet this is a crucial time for you too. A time when your body needs to recover. Generally, we talk about the postnatal period lasting for about six weeks after the birth, but for most mothers, the recovery period may be nine months to a year. While you may be keen to get back to exercising you must give yourself some breathing space. This is true even if you had a straightforward normal delivery. If you had a difficult delivery or a caesarean section you will need to be patient until you have been given the all clear by your medical practitioner.

In the meantime, chances are you are not getting much sleep! For all new mothers it is essential that you put some time aside to look after yourself and relax. It's a good idea to get your partner to do some relaxation exercises too! It's surprising how sensitive babies can be to their parents' moods. If they feel you are tired or stressed, they can become fractious too! It's in both your interests to keep your energy and spirits up. A few minutes each day to do some very gentle exercise can release those feel-good endorphins and make all the difference. It is sound advice to take things easy for the first six weeks at least.

Looking back over the previous chapters you can see the multitude of ways in which your body changed as the pregnancy progressed. You had months to adjust to these changes. Now, however, after the birth, your body is changing again, but even more rapidly. Let's look more closely at some of these changes.

Your changing body

With the birth of your baby you now no longer carry the combined weight of the baby, placenta, amniotic fluid and membranes. This means that your centre of gravity changes quite literally overnight. Once again, this means that your posture adapts. You might have trouble with your balance as your body is not used to its new posture yet. It may be some time before you return to your pre-pregnancy posture, if at all.

Ligamentous laxity can continue to affect your joints for months after the birth. If you are breastfeeding it will affect you longer as your body continues to produce the pregnancy hormones. We will need to be cautious in our choice of exercise, avoid overstretching, wide ranges of movement, single leg weight bearing as before and focus instead on lots of spinal and pelvic stability exercises.

Unfortunately, caring for a baby involves a lot of bending, lifting, and twisting which may place a strain on all your vulnerable joints. If you are breastfeeding the neck and upper shoulders are going to still be affected by the weight of the breasts and by sitting for long periods feeding. Try to feed the baby before you do your exercises as your breasts will be more comfortable if they are less full. Of course, if you are bottle-feeding you still have to sit still and hold the baby so you may still get neck and shoulder pain. Add to this the strain of having to carry the baby and all the baby's paraphernalia around with you. Therefore, exercises which open out your upper body, releasing tension, will be high on our priority list, but you are also going to need to work on your upper body strength.

Meanwhile, the rest of your body may still be showing the after-effects of the pregnancy. Your waist may still appear thicker, your thighs and bottom a little flabbier than normal. Do not worry, we will be targeting these areas in the workouts. Fortunately the puffiness in your feet and ankles will disappear quite soon as most women sweat out the excess fluid they gained during pregnancy.

With your baby born, the uterus can return to its normal size. This will happen gradually and is known as involution. If you are breastfeeding, you may even feel your uterus squeezing as your baby suckles. This is because when the baby sucks it stimulates the release of the hormone oxytocin, which not only stimulates milk flow but also your uterus to contract. The pains usually last just a few days and are accompanied by a discharge known as lochia, which is the shedding of the lining of the uterus. The uterus usually takes about six weeks to return to its normal size. To help, as soon as you can, you can try some gentle pelvic tilting in the form of Pelvic Tilts (page 197) not coming up high, just the initial action of tipping the pelvis back. You can also try lying on your front with some pillows under your hips. The pillows will tilt your pelvis encouraging all the internal organs to resume their normal positions.

Ribcage changes

We noted before how your ribcage elevates during pregnancy. The circumference of your chest increases by up to 7cm and does not always return to normal after the delivery. We are going to have to work on this. Key to helping the ribs come back down is working on your oblique muscles.

With this in mind we have created the image of 'The X Factor'! Visualise a big 'X' on your trunk connecting the ribs on one side to the hip on the other side. It's an imaginary 'X' and it adds another dimension to your core.

We may cue you to connect just one half of the X Factor, connecting rib to opposite hip. This helps with your stability. See page 58.

Try also the following experiment. Sit tall and place your hands on your ribs. Breathe in and as you breathe out make a loud shhhhhing noise... feel your ribs drawing down and together.

You can use this if you like while doing some of the exercises to help connect your ribs… shhhing would be good with Spine Curls with Flies for example.

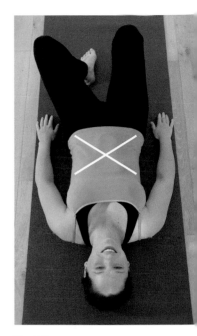

The X Factor

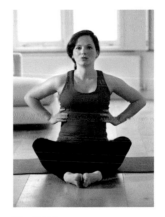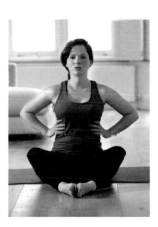

The Shhhh

> **Medical permission**
> As with the antenatal exercise programme, only your medical practitioner knows your medical history well enough to decide when it is safe for you to start exercising again. Do ask for their consent. On page 212 there is a list of contraindications to postnatal exercise.

The pelvic floor

If you had a vaginal delivery, your perineum is probably going to feel sore after the delivery. The pressure of the baby's head passing though the vagina will probably have bruised the area and you may have stitches from a tear or an episiotomy (a cut sometimes made to enlarge the vagina opening during delivery). This may have been aggravated if there was any medical intervention such the use of forceps.

You will probably feel the need to empty your bladder frequently as your body rids itself of the extra fluid you carried during pregnancy. If you had an epidural during labour then you may have had a catheter fitted to help, and you may not yet have normal sensation in that region. It is possible that you will find passing urine difficult and you may also suffer from stress incontinence – where you will pass urine involuntarily whenever extra pressure is created inside the abdomen, for example when you cough or sneeze. If you did your pelvic floor exercises regularly throughout your pregnancy you will be less likely to suffer from this.

If you had a caesarean section you should carry on doing your pelvic floor exercises, as your baby still used your pelvic floor as a trampoline for the last few months. Whichever type of delivery you had, the last thing you probably feel like doing at this stage is pelvic floor exercises – you may imagine that they will aggravate the stitches, but in fact the opposite is true. These exercises tighten and relax the muscles and thus encourage the flow of blood to the area, which helps the healing process and reduces any swelling. You should start your pelvic floor exercises 24 hours after the birth. You can do all the pelvic floor exercises we have already given you: the Wind Zip, the Pelvic Elevator, the Emergency Stop, the Pillow Squeeze, the Abdominal Breathing exercise for Release and the Flower.

We have added some more, yes more, to the Postnatal Programme such as the Standing Pelvic Floor Exercises on page 210 – we never give up! It is very useful to practise your pelvic floor exercises in a variety of positions as some positions are more challenging than others.

If you think about it, engaging your pelvic floor during a Spine Curl for example is relatively easy as gravity is helping you, but keeping your pelvic floor engaged when standing is altogether more demanding. Add a few extra movements on to distract you, and you'll find it even harder. But, in the real world, this is what it is like. Chances are you are going to need to engage your pelvic floor to stop yourself passing urine, while say, doing the shopping or lifting your baby. It is much more likely that you will need these muscles while out and about than while sitting quietly on a chair or lying on a mat! Lifting and carrying the baby and equipment places extra strain on your pelvic floor so it helps to train your muscles.

Mood changes

It is perfectly normal for you to experience mood changes after the birth, blame those hormones once again. Add to this lack of sleep or disturbed sleep! It may be that you feel very low, or very high or that you swing between the two. It is very common to feel an abrupt drop in mood and a sudden feeling of depression. 'Baby blues' is a mild type of depression that occurs after childbirth, usually around the third to the tenth day after giving birth. It can last from a few hours to a few days. During this time you may feel tearful and irritable. 'Baby blues' is said to be experienced by more than half of all mothers in the western world. You may be surprised to know that men can be affected too. The birth of a new baby can be stressful for both parents and some fathers feel unable to cope, or feel they are not giving their partner the support she needs. They can also find it difficult to adjust to the big changes and demands made by a new baby.

Sometimes this feeling of depression does not pass and may become severe. Research suggests that postnatal depression affects about 1 in 10 women. In fact these figures may only reflect the tip of the iceberg, the figure has been thought to be nearer 1 in 7 or even 1 in 5.

If you feel that you need some extra help, do speak to your doctor. He may ask you some simple questions such as, have you been experiencing:

– disturbed sleep
– tearfulness
– problems concentrating or making decisions
– low self-confidence
– a loss of appetite or an increased appetite (comfort eating is often a symptom of depression)
– feeling anxious
– having panic attacks
– feeling tired, listless and reluctant to undertake any physical activity
– feeling guilty or self-critical
– feeling as if you cannot cope
– suicidal thoughts.

Sometimes, a doctor may do a blood test to make sure there is not a physical reason for symptoms like tiredness and low mood, such as an underactive thyroid gland or anaemia. These conditions often occur after having a baby. Depending on your responses to the above, your doctor may ask if you would like some professional help. Go to the back of the book for some useful websites.

Caesarean births

If you had a caesarean birth you must remember that you have undergone major abdominal surgery and this will affect your ability to exercise.

Your operation may have been planned well in advance (elective) or it may have been an emergency decision taken because your labour was not progressing and the baby, or yourself, were becoming distressed.

If it was an elective caesarean, you will have been well prepared and the whole process was, hopefully, ordered and calm. If it was an emergency operation, however, you will probably be feeling exhausted and somewhat bruised by the experience. You may have gone through a difficult first stage of labour. Do give yourself extra time to rest and heal.

In either case, you will find that for the first few days you will be uncomfortable because of the incision scar. Moving about will be difficult. Your pelvic floor will be less traumatised by the birth, but will still have been stretched by your pregnancy, so it is important to start pelvic floor exercises as soon as your practitioner gives you the go-ahead. Connecting to your core muscles may feel strange at first but do persevere.

You may find yourself stooping as you are afraid of the pain and you try to protect the scar and stitches. This is a natural reaction but you should try to stand tall. Use your breathing to help you relax. You can gently support your abdomen with your hand and use core connection to give you extra support.

Whenever you are getting on or off the bed, try to avoid awkward twisting movements or sitting straight up quickly. Someone should help you. Bend your knees and keeping them together roll onto your side. Then, carefully push yourself up into sitting allowing your legs to swing over the side of the bed and onto the floor. If the bed is at the right height you can then stand up easily. If not, ask for the bed to be adjusted.

To get back into bed sit on the edge as near to the head of the bed as possible and zipping up, lift your legs one at a time onto the bed. If necessary lift your legs with your hands. Then with the knees still bent, dig your heels into the mattress and lower yourself back towards the head of the bed with your hands.

Ask your practitioner if you may try the following simple exercises. You may need to wait a few days.

Circulation exercises

Your circulation will be affected so it is important that you start to get the blood flowing again. At first you will have to practise these on the bed, but eventually you can do them on the exercise mat.

Sit tall on your bed, with your back well supported by pillows. Have your legs out in front of you hip-width apart, parallel but ensure that your knees are softly bent.

1 Breathing normally, point and flex your feet about 10 times. Pause, then do another 6 repetitions.

2 Take your feet a little wider apart now, still breathing normally, and with control circle your ankles 6 times in each direction.

3 Lying on your bed in the Relaxation Position do slow and controlled Leg Slides as described on page 58. Repeat 6 times with each leg.

Breathing exercise

If you had a general anaesthetic, then you should add the following exercise which will help to clear any secretions in the lungs left as a result of the anaesthetic. If they linger in the lungs you risk infection and, for obvious reasons, you will not be too keen on coughing at the moment, which would be the natural way to get rid of them.

1 Sit tall in your bed or on a sturdy chair (the key is to lengthen up through the spine as you will find it hard to breathe with bad posture because your ribcage is closed down).

2 Place one hand onto your scar to give it gentle support.

3 Breathe in wide and full and allow your ribs to expand – think of nappy bucket handles lifting.

4 As you breathe out, focus on completely wringing out the lungs, make a 'huffing' noise to help, think of the bucket handles closing back down. Make sure you fully empty your lungs and relax the ribcage, allowing the breastbone to soften.

Repeat 8 times. Try to do this 5 times a day. Eventually you can add your Wind Zip.

Getting back to exercise after a caesarean section

Your recovery is going to take several weeks. You must not do any heavy lifting, other than your baby, for at least 6 weeks. You should have a follow-up consultation with your surgeon, this will give you the perfect opportunity to ask if you are ready to exercise again.

If you are given permission to start exercising again, try the simple exercises listed on pages 212–213. Do not attempt any Curl Ups or similar strong abdominal exercises for about five months. We want the scar tissue to heal first.

Postnatal weight loss: getting back to normal

Naturally, you will have lost some weight immediately following the birth. You will also lose some of the puffiness over the next few weeks as new mothers perspire a lot to help get rid of excess fluid in the body. But how long is it going to take you to return to your pre-pregnant weight?

A lot of new mothers worry about this. It depends on a wide variety of factors including how much weight you gained, your levels of activity, whether you are breastfeeding. Mothers report that it can take between six weeks and six months to go back to their pre-pregnancy weight. Some mothers claim that they never get back to it!

The most important thing is that you do not compare yourself to other new mothers. Keeping your energy levels up and staying healthy is far more important than rushing to get your figure back. Some books claim that breastfeeding will help weight loss. While it certainly means that you are using up lots of extra calories, it is important at the same time that you consume extra calories to keep your milk flowing and it also means that some of the pregnancy hormones are still present.

All through the book we have been talking about keeping a balance and the same is true here. Of course you want your old figure back, and our exercise programme will help you to achieve this, but for the next few months, while your body is recovering, you need to avoid dieting and strenuous exercise.

Postnatal commonly asked questions

Question: **I had a lot of pain in the front of my pelvis in the last two months of my pregnancy, and although it is a lot better now I have had the baby, I still get sharp pains especially when I get in and out of the bath. Why am I still getting pain and what can I do about it?**

Pelvic girdle pain is common during and after pregnancy, affecting as many as 1 in 5 women. The pain can start as early as the first trimester, or it may only occur in the latter stages as the baby's head engages. The symptoms can be varied and include pubic pain, inner thigh and groin pain, back, sacrum, buttock and hip pain and are often aggravated by walking, climbing steps or stairs, turning over in bed and activities that involve standing on one leg (for example putting a sock on).

As we saw on page 17, the pregnancy hormones can cause the ligaments that bind the pelvic bones together to become more elastic. These hormones may continue to affect you for several months after the birth. The pain frequently arises as a result of a minor displacement at the front of the pelvis, leading to an increase in the normal gap between the pubic joints. This is termed symphysis pubis dysfunction (SPD). An overstretch at this joint can cause joint strain in the other pelvic girdle joints, such as the sacroiliac joints.

Although this can be a debilitating condition, it can be well managed with a specific progressive exercise programme to increase the support offered by the soft tissues around the pelvis. The Pilates exercises in this book offer a perfect choice of such exercises, but in acutely painful cases, it may be relevant to exercise under the supervision of a professional such as a physiotherapist, chiropractor or osteopath. Your GP may refer you to a manual therapist as small pelvic adjustments may be required to aid with pain relief. Your manual therapist will also encourage you to practise specific exercises to improve pelvic stability.

A pelvic support belt (e.g. a Serola belt) may also be used to assist the pelvic stability. The belts are discreet, and there is a maternity option offering bump support in addition.

Avoidance of aggravating activities is also encouraged, for example you may try walking with a smaller stride length. Take care not to do any exercises which require you to take your weight onto one leg or where you put pressure on the pubic bone. Side-lying exercises may also prove uncomfortable until you feel better. If you have any doubts about pelvic pain during labour, your midwife will be able to suggest alternative birthing positions.

For more information about pelvic girdle pain and pelvic support belts, check Further Information (page 223).

Question: **Help! My baby is 9 months old but my abdominal divide is still 3cm and I'm still doming when I do a Curl Up.**

Even though you are now 9 months postnatal, it is still important to refer to the section on diastasis recti, and follow the advice given, starting with the early abdominal exercise programme, and progressing through the exercises as advised. Don't be tempted to progress too quickly to the more challenging exercises, as this may further delay your recovery. If you have concerns, your GP may refer you to an obstetric physiotherapist for further advice.

Diastasis Recti

We have noted all through the book how your abdominal muscles will stretch and separate to accommodate your growing baby. In most cases the two sides come together spontaneously after six weeks, but sometimes they do not always knit back together on their own sufficiently. Sometimes they need some help.

Why is it important to help improve the diastasis?
Apart from the divide and bulge not looking very flattering, we must also remember the vital role that your abdominals play in the stability of your pelvis and spine and in good movement and posture. You may be more prone to back problems if your diastasis remains large. In severe cases, you may get a herniation, which may need surgery to repair.

How do you know whether your abdominals have mended properly or not?
Your healthcare practitioner may do The Rectus Check for you at your postnatal check-up. Many mothers, however, seem to miss out on this.

The test is very simple and can be done easily yourself. You can do the check a few weeks after the birth (wait longer if you have had a difficult birth or a caesarean section).

If you feel a significant divide, that is more than 2cm or 2 fingers-width) or if you notice any doming or bulging along the divide when doing the test, then follow the exercise programme on page 212 and check again each week. Avoid doing normal Curl Up-style exercises (that is those which involve trunk flexion) until the divide reduces to less than 2cm and there's no doming.

It can take many months for the divide to improve. Sometimes, it can remain for years. If you are concerned about the divide, you may consult your medical practitioner who may refer you to a physiotherapist for a more intensive rehabilitation plan.

Diastasis recti

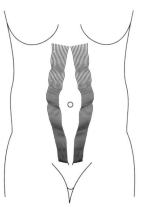

<table>
<tr><td>

To help correct a diastasis recti...
You will need to focus on three main things:
1. Pelvic Tilts (baby Spine Curls)
2. Pelvic Stability exercises, in particular exercises where the trunk stays still but the abdominals are working!
3. Assisted Curl Ups with towel.
All of these are covered in the Postnatal Programme.

</td></tr>
</table>

The 'Rec Check'

Note that the divide may be behind, below or above the navel (or even the whole length) so you will need to check each section.

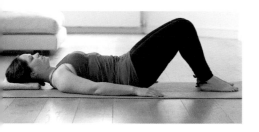

Starting position...

Lie in the Relaxation Position.

Find your navel with your hand, placing two fingers widthways as shown. Be firm with the pressure.

Note: if you feel any strain in your neck doing this, you may support your head with one hand (as if about to do a Curl Up).

Action...

1 Breathe in to prepare.

2 Breathe out as you nod your head and curl the upper body from the mat. At the same time press your two fingers into your navel.

3 Notice what has happened to the divide under your fingertips

Can you feel the two edges of your rectus abdominis muscle?

Is this gap more than two fingers-width, 2cm?

Is there any doming or bulging?

4 Breathe in and roll back down with control.

5 Now, slide your fingers up from the navel along the centre line about 4cm. Locate the divide once more and repeat the Curl Up, noting what happens again.

6 Lastly, repeat the test again but this time have your fingers a few centimetres below the navel (obviously avoid this part if you've had a caesarean section).

If the gap was 2 fingers-width, or less, and if there was no doming or bulging, your abdominals are mending nicely and you may proceed with the normal postnatal exercises and workouts on page 212–213.

If you felt a significant gap of more than 2cm or noticed doming, then follow the programme below and check again in a week's time to see if there is a difference. In the meantime, avoid any Curl Up type exercises, other than Assisted Curl Ups on page 206.

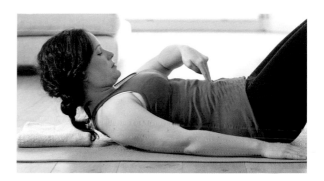

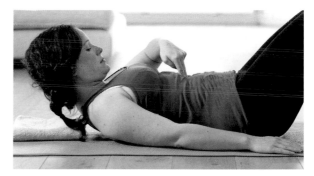

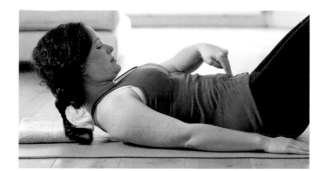

The Postnatal Programme

This programme has been designed specifically to help get you back in shape and particularly to improve your abdominal integrity. It is thus perfect to help improve a diastasis recti.

If you are joining us here and are new to Pilates you will need to learn the basics of Pilates. If you have taken a break from Pilates, then revisiting the basics would be a good idea too. Practise the following exercises from The Fundamentals.

Alignment

Posture Check . . . . *(page 137)*

Wall Slides A or B . . . . *(pages 36–39)*

Relaxation Position . . . . *(pages 40–41)*

Compass . . . . *(pages 42–43)*

Seated on a Mat (Long Frog) . . . . *(page 44)*

Seated on a Chair . . . . *(page 45)*

Avoid Four-point Kneeling for the first few weeks
      postnatal . . . . *(pages 46–47)*

High Kneeling . . . . *(page 48)*

Prone . . . . *(page 49)*

Side-lying (caution if you have pelvic girdle pain)   *(page 50)*

Standing . . . . *(page 53)*

Pilates Stance . . . . *(page 52)*

Neck Rolls, Chin Tucks . . . . *(pages 54–55)*

Breathing

Scarf Breathing . . . . *(page 56)*

Centring

Wind Zip . . . . *(page 60)*

Leg Slides . . . . *(page 62)*

Knee Openings (care if you have had a C section) *(page 63)*

Single Knee Folds (NOT Double) . . . . *(page 63)*

Floating Arms . . . . *(page 66)*

Ribcage Closure . . . . *(page 68)*

Starfish . . . . *(page 70)*

Spine Curls (try Spine Curls with Support first,
      page 199) . . . . *(page 72)*

The Postnatal exercises

Check your posture on a regular basis, and include the appropriate Wall Slide to help improve it (see page 210).

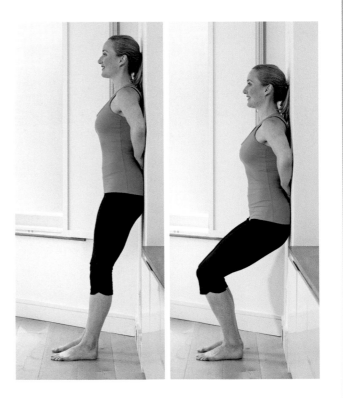

Pelvic Tilts

This is essentially just rolling the pelvis to North in a baby Spine Curl. *Suitable for...* Preparation for Pregnancy, Early Pregnancy and Postnatal.

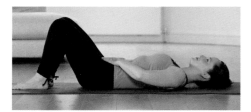

Starting position...

The Relaxation Position. Place your hands on your pelvis for reference.
Zip up to maintain a constant and appropriate connection to your centre throughout.

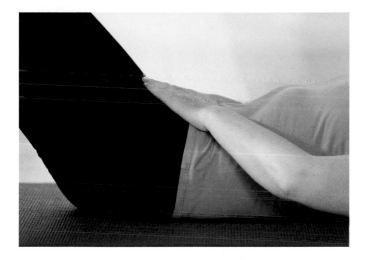 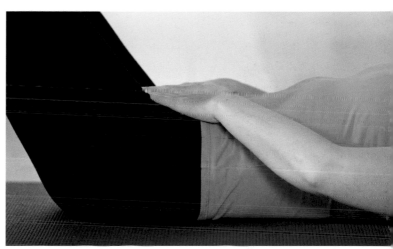

Action...

1   Breathe in to prepare.

2   Breathe out as you tilt your pelvis backwards, your tailbone curls under, your pubic bone moves back, the whole pelvis rolls on the thigh bones. It's a small movement.

3   Breathe in and release the pelvis back to neutral with control.
Repeat *up to 10 times.*

✳ **Watchpoints**
–   Ensure equal weight through both feet – this will help to avoid your pelvis dipping to either side.
–   Keep the waist equally long on both sides.
–   Keep the knees parallel, in line with your hips, and avoid your feet rolling in or out.

Pelvic Stability Exercises

Any of the following exercises would be appropriate: Leg Slides; Knee Openings; Single Knee Folds; Oyster; Starfish.

What we would like you to focus on in addition to your normal core connection is the 'X Factor' connection. Looking at Knee Openings, for example – as your right knee opens, think of connecting your right rib to your left hip. This should help with your stability.

As your left knee opens, think of connecting your left rib to your right hip.

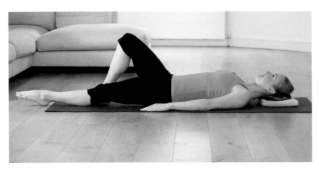

Leg Slides *See page 62*

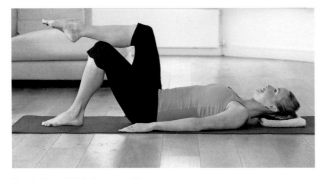

Single Knee Folds *See page 63*

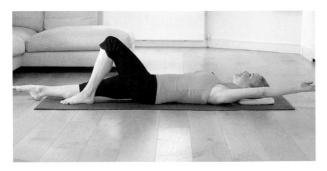

Starfish *See page 70*

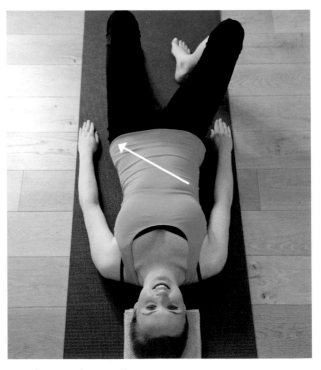

Knee Openings *See page 63*

Spine Curls with Support (scarf and cushion)

This variation is the one to choose when you start back with your Pilates practice. The scarf and cushion give you additional support and a sense of security. *Suitable for...* Preparing for Pregnancy, Early Pregnancy, Postnatal. **Equipment** A scarf or stretchband and small cushion.

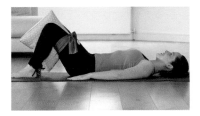

Starting position...

The Relaxation Position. Wrap a scarf around your thighs and place a small pillow between your knees. Your arms are lengthened down by the side of your body. **Zip up to maintain a constant and appropriate connection to your centre throughout.**

Action...

1 Breathe in to prepare your body to move.

2 Breathe out as you curl your tailbone under, imprinting your lower back into the mat before beginning to peel your spine off the mat one vertebra at a time. Roll your spine sequentially, bone by bone to the tips of the shoulder-blades.

3 Breathe in and hold this position, focusing on the length in your spine.

4 Breathe out as you roll the spine back down, softening the breastbone and wheeling once again, every single bone gets its turn.

5 Breathe in as you release the pelvis back to level again.

Repeat *up to 10 times.*

✳ Watchpoints

– Focus on wheeling your spine off the mat vertebra by vertebra.

– Control the sequential return of your spine back down to the mat.

– Avoid rolling up too far, maintain a connection of your ribs to your pelvis and avoid arching your spine.

– Ensure equal weight through both feet; this will help to avoid your pelvis dipping to either side.

– Try to avoid 'hitching' your pelvis up towards your ribcage, keep the waist equally long on both sides.

– Keep the knees parallel, in line with your hips, and avoid your feet rolling in or out.

– Allow your collar-bones to widen and keep the neck long and free from tension.

Spine Curls with Arm Flies

This version has the added benefit of helping to close your ribs. Revise the shhhing noise on page 189. *Suitable for...* Preparing for Pregnancy, Early Pregnancy, Postnatal.

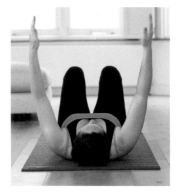

Starting position...
The Relaxation Position, arms raised above your shoulders in a Shoulder Drop position, palms facing inwards.

Watchpoints As before plus:
- Visualise your ribs closing down as you shhhhh.
- Move the arms from the shoulder joints only.
- Your open arms should stay lengthened but keep a soft bend in the elbows.
- Your open arms may touch the floor, but should not rest there.
- As your arms close back in, keep the collar-bones open.

Action...
1 Breathe out and Spine Curl and zip up as before.
2 At the height of the curl, breathe in and open both arms out to the sides.

3 Breathe out and, as you Spine Curl back down, slowly close your arms back to the starting position. Make the shhhhing noise as you do so. **Repeat** *up to 10 times.*

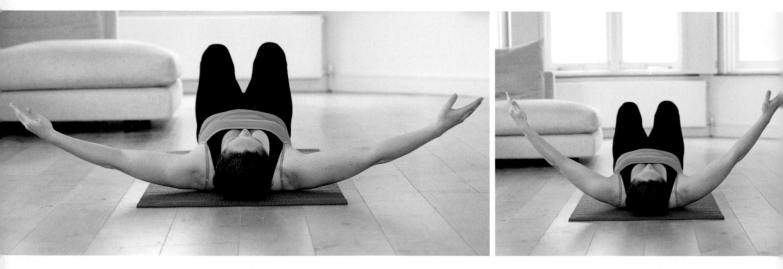

Spine Curls with Knee Openings

This version is more challenging so should be saved until you feel stronger. It combines segmental control of the spine with additional pelvic stability. *Suitable for...* Preparing for Pregnancy. Postnatal only after about 8 weeks when you are feeling back to normal.

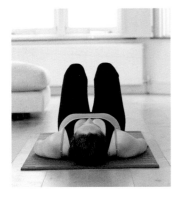

Starting position...

Relaxation Position.

Zip up to maintain a constant and appropriate connection to your centre throughout.

Action...

1 Breathe in to prepare.

2 Breathe out as you Spine Curl up but this time do not go quite so high.

3 Breathe in and hold the position.

4 Breathe out and slowly with control open one knee to the side. Do not disturb your pelvis, it must stay still.

5 Breathe in and return the knee.

6 Repeat with the other knee. Check that you have kept your pelvis lifted and steady.

7 Breathe out and roll back down bone by bone.

Repeat *up to 4 times.*

Ribcage Closure and Leg Slides

A fun combination of two exercises that feels really good as you stretch out from your strong centre. *Suitable for...* Preparing for Pregnancy, Early Pregnancy, Postnatal.

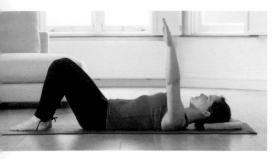

Starting position...

The Relaxation Position, lengthen your arms by the side of your body on the mat. **Zip up to maintain a constant and appropriate connection to your centre throughout.**

✳ Watchpoints

– Remember that your arms may not reach the floor, do not force them back.

– During the exhalation, focus on the closing and softening of the ribcage.

– Keep your neck long and free from tension; your head remains still and heavy throughout.

– Focus on your waist remaining long and even on both sides as you slide your leg in and out.

– Keep your foot in contact with the floor and in a line with your hip.

Action...

1 Breathe in and raise both arms to shoulder height, palms facing forwards.

2 Breathe out as you reach both arms overhead towards the floor, simultaneously slide one leg away along the mat in line with your hip. Your ribs stay connected, your pelvis and spine undisturbed.

3 Breathe in as you return the arms above your chest and draw the leg back to the Starting position.

4 Repeat, sliding the other leg.

Repeat *the sequence 3 times, then lengthen the arms back down alongside your body.*

Postnatal Pelvic Stability Exercises

This series of exercises is designed to help knit those abdominals together again and improve your stability. If you have been following the Antenatal Programme you will already be familiar with some of the movements, now we are going to put those skills to the test!

Arms Raised: Leg Slides, Single Knee Folds, Knee Openings, Knee Circles

Revise the directions for Leg Slides (see page 62), Single Knee Folds (*not* double) (see page 63), Knee Openings and Circles (see pages 63, 120) *Suitable for...* Preparing for Pregnancy, Early Pregnancy, Postnatal.

Starting position...

For all the above

The Relaxation Position, raise both arms to shoulder height, palms facing forwards.

Action...

1 Layer your 'X Factor' over your zip! For example, if you are folding your right knee in, think of connecting your right rib to your left hip. If you are folding your left knee in, connect left rib to right hip. It is the same with Leg Slides, Knee Openings, Knee Circles.

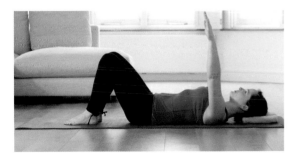

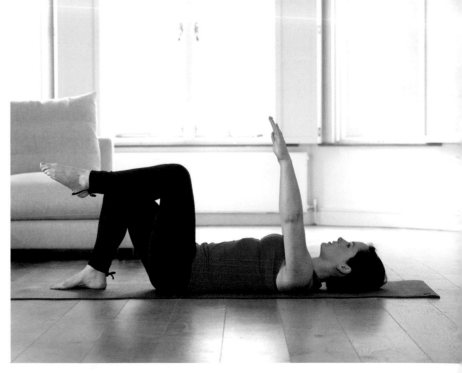

> **✳ Watchpoints**
>
> *Refer to the relevant Watchpoints for each movement, but focus particularly on:*
>
> – Not holding your breath
> – Keeping your waist long and even on both sides
> – Keeping your pelvis still and stable
> – Keeping your chest and front of your shoulders open. If you feel tension creeping in, stop and do a few Shoulder Drops (page 80) before continuing.

Arms raised with bilateral band pull:
Leg Slides, Single Knee Folds, Knee Openings, Knee Circles

For these variations, we have added an extra element which should help you feel your abdominals engage even more. For Leg Slides (see page 62), Single Knee Folds (*not* double) – see page 63, Knee Openings and Circles (see pages 63, 120) *Suitable for...* Postnatal. **Equipment** stretch band or stretchy scarf.

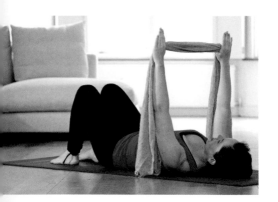

✳ Watchpoints *As before plus:*

– Keep your wrists lengthened and in good alignment. Notice how the band is held with lengthened wrist and long fingers.

– Keep your collar bones open.

– You will have to be vigilant in not allowing tension to creep into the shoulders. If you feel this happening stop and do some Shoulder Drops.

Starting position...

The Relaxation Position. Holding the band, raise both arms to shoulder height, palms facing forwards.

Action...

1 You are going to follow all the directions as before, but this time you should maintain a constant but gentle pull on the band/scarf with your arms. It is important that you pull evenly on both sides. Visualise your abdominals: the deep layers, the 'X Factor', all knitting together. Remember, if you are sliding your right leg away think of connecting your right rib to your left hip. If you are sliding your left leg away, connect left rib to right hip. Ditto Knee Folds, Knee Openings , Knee Circles.

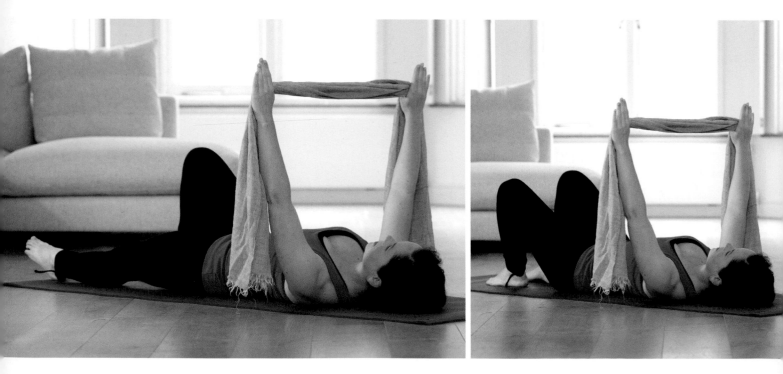

Arms raised with unilateral band pull:

Leg Slides, Single Knee Folds, Knee Openings, Knee Circles This version is more challenging as you have to use your core muscles to stay centred and stable as you pull on the band with one arm, while working the opposite leg. This creates a diagonal pull across the torso. Feel your abdominals wrap automatically around your trunk to keep you stable! For Leg Slides (see page 62), Single Knee Folds (*not* Double) – see page 63, Knee Openings and Circles (see pages 63, 120) *Suitable for...* Postnatal. **Equipment** stretch band or stretchy scarf.

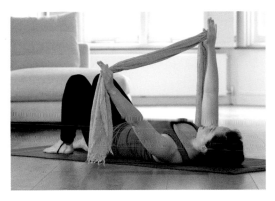

Action...

Follow all the directions as before. Holding the band, raise both arms to shoulder height, palms facing forwards, but this time you should maintain a constant but gentle pull on the band/scarf with just one arm, not both. Then you are going to Leg Slide, Knee Open, Single Knee Fold or Knee Circle with the opposite leg. Once again visualise your abdominals: the deep layers, the 'X Factor', all knitting together.

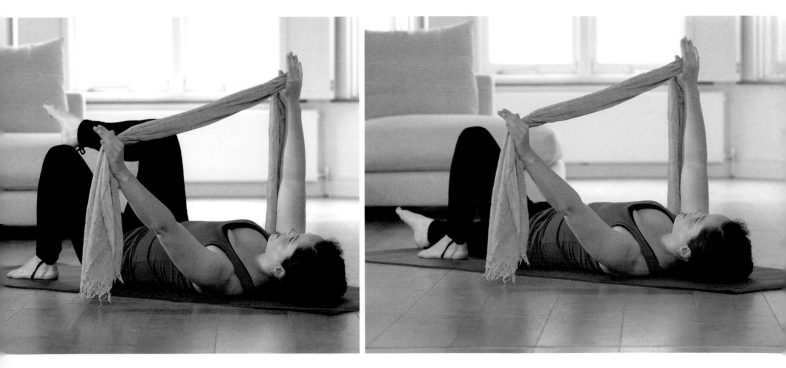

Assisted Curl Ups

Remember this is the only Curl Up recommended until the diastasis improves. The idea is that the towel will help to pull the two sides of the muscle together again. *Suitable for...* Postnatal. **Note** Unlike our normal Curl Ups, in this version you are not supporting your head with your hands. Take extra care that you do not strain your neck. We have suggested that you have a flat cushion or towel under your head. Remember to nod the head first then sequentially roll up. Stop if you feel any strain in your neck. Go back and practise Pelvic Tilts and Stability exercises until you feel stronger. You can always try a bigger cushion under the head too. **Equipment** A large towel (do not use a stretch band as it will give too much). A flat cushion or folded towel for under your head.

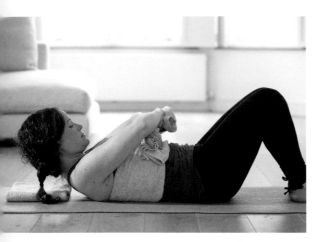 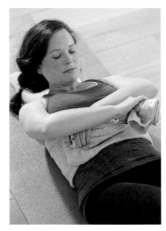

* Watchpoints
- Ensure that your pelvis remains grounded in neutral throughout; curl up only as far as this can be maintained.
- Although your pelvis remains still, the natural curve in your lower spine will open out and release into the mat.
- Keep pulling, pulling, pulling on the towel. Visualise the two sides of your abdominals knitting together.

Starting position...

Lay the towel onto the mat widthways so that when you lie down it will wrap around your midriff. Come into the Relaxation Position. Place the other towel or flat cushion under your head. Now cross your arms so that each hand takes hold of the opposite edge of the towel.

Zip up to maintain a constant and appropriate connection to your centre throughout.

Action...

1 Breathe in, preparing your body to move.

2 Breathe out as you nod your head and sequentially curl up the upper body, keeping the back of your lower ribcage in contact with the mat. Simultaneously pull the two sides of the towel together. Squeeze, squeeze, squeeze…

3 Breathe in to the back of your ribcage and maintain the curled up position.

4 Breathe out as you slowly curl back down, keeping pulling on the towel until you have fully returned on the mat. Breathe in and release.

Repeat *up to 10 times.*

Cobra Prep

At last you can lie on your front! Most baby-caring activities involve bending forwards so you will want to include lots of back extension exercises like Diamond Press, Star, Dart and now a new one, Cobra Prep. *Suitable for...* Preparing for Pregnancy, Early Pregnancy, Postnatal.

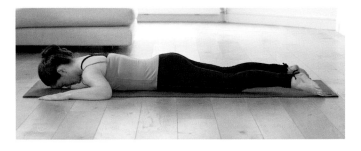

Starting position...

Lie on your front, rest your forehead on the mat or a folded towel. Your legs are straight, slightly wider than hip-width and turned out from the hips. Bend your elbows and position your hands slightly wider than and above your shoulders, your palms are facing down. Make sure that your shoulders are released and your collar-bones are wide.

Zip up to maintain a constant and appropriate connection to your centre throughout.

Action...

1 Breathe in to prepare your body to move.

2 Breathe out as you longthen the front of the neck to roll and lift your head, then chest off the mat. Your arms will begin to straighten slightly. Your lower ribs remain in contact with the mat, but open your chest and focus on directing it forwards.

3 Breathe in as you hold this lengthened and lifted position.

4 Breathe out as you return your chest and head sequentially back down to the mat, allowing the arms to bend back to the Starting position.

Repeat *up to 10 times. Then, unless you are doing another prone exercise, come back into Rest Position.*

* Watchpoints

– Start the movement by lengthening and lifting your head first, and then your neck.

– Keep your abdominals gently connected to support your spine.

– Avoid too much pressure into the arms; they are there to lightly support you, not to press you up.

Crawling Lizard

Here is another back extension exercise which is a little bit different in that it 'mimics' the action that your baby will try when they are getting ready to crawl. They may even copy you if they watch you doing it. *Suitable for...* Preparing for Pregnancy, Early Pregnancy, Postnatal.

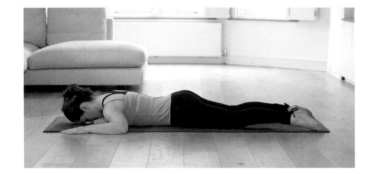

Starting position...

Lie on your front in a straight line and rest your forehead on the mat or a folded towel. Your legs are straight, slightly wider than hip-width and turned out from the hips. Bend your elbows and position your hands slightly wider than, and above, your shoulders. Your palms are facing down. Make sure that your shoulders are released and your collar-bones are wide.

Zip up to maintain a constant and appropriate connection to your centre throughout..

Action...

1 Breathe in as you lengthen the front of the neck to roll and lift your head until it is in line with your spine

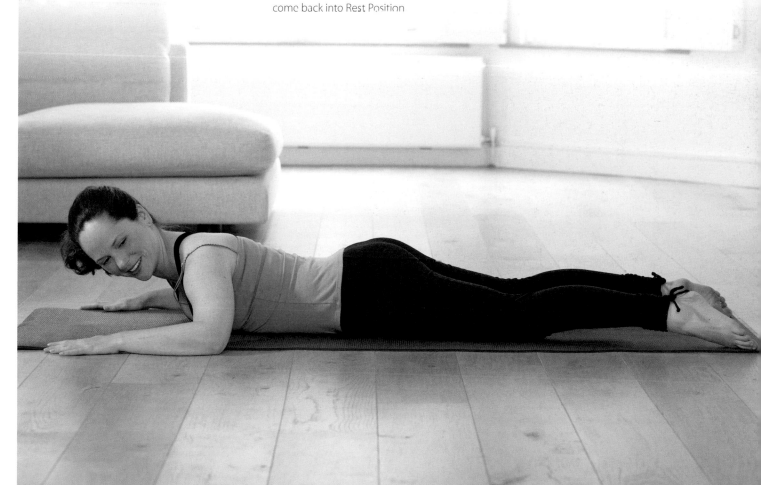

2   Breathe out as you open your left shoulder pressing gently on your left hand, rotating your ribs to the left until you are looking over your left shoulder.

3   Breathe into that open side and hold the position.

4   Breathe out and slowly return to the starting position, moving first through your ribs, shoulder and finally bringing your head back to rest.

5   Repeat with the right side.

Repeat the sequence up to 4 times. Then, unless you are doing another prone exercise, come back into Rest Position

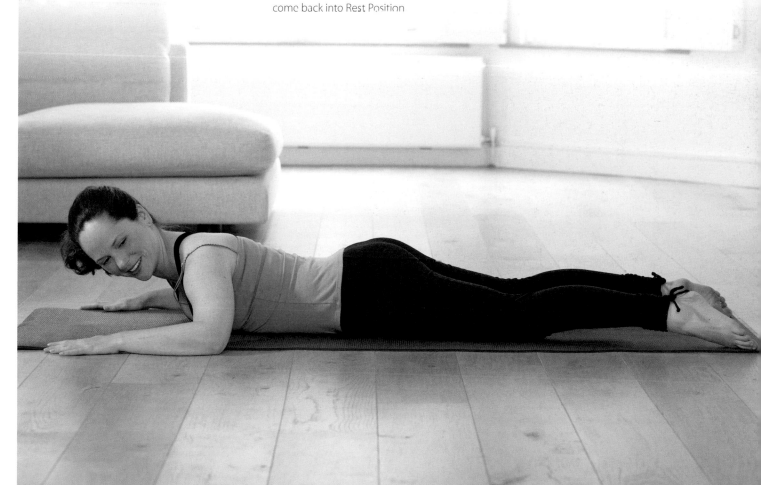

Standing Pelvic Floor Exercises

Lots of variations to play with. While eventually we want to train your muscles to hold a full bladder, you may be kind to yourself and empty your bladder first. When you think you have enough control, try it with a fuller bladder.

Wall Slides

Wall Slide Position (see pages 36–39). Engage your pelvic floor as if trying to prevent passing wind and water (all we need is earth and fire!) as you slide up and down the wall three times, then release. Keep breathing.

Standing

Stand tall on the floor (see page 53). Engage your pelvic floor as above. You can always then add an arm movement such as Floating Arms or Dumb Waiter to challenge your concentration, and ability to control your pelvic floor while distracted.

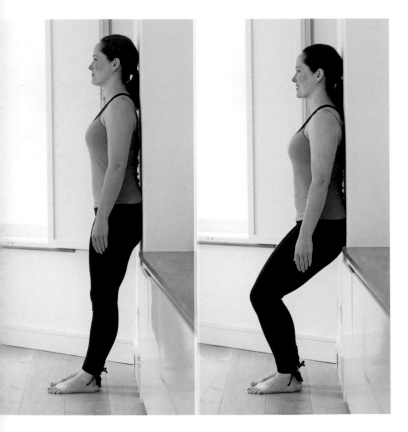

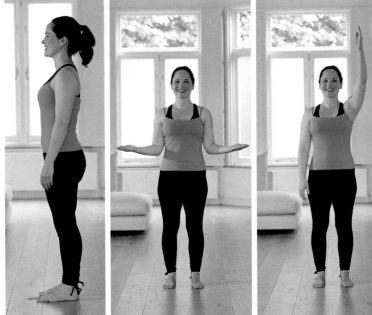

Pilates Stance

Stand tall in Pilates Stance (see page 52). Engage your pelvic floor as above. Then add an arm movement such as Floating Arms or Dumb Waiter as before.

Pilates Wide-leg Stance

Wide-leg Pilates Stance. Legs turned out from your hips. Follow the directions as above. The hardest one of all. Now come up on your toes... bring your pelvic floor with you!

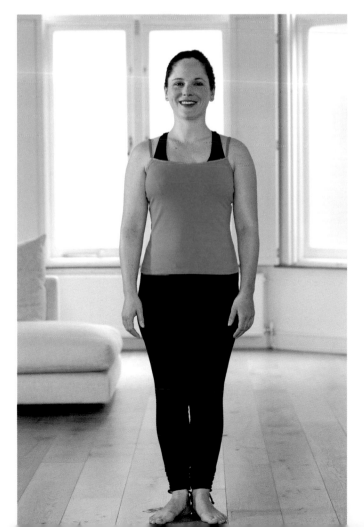

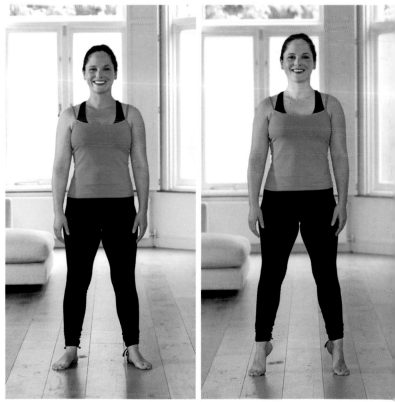

Postnatal Workouts

In addition to the exercises demonstrated in this chapter, the following exercises from the rest of the book will also be helpful.

From Preparing for Pregnancy

Pelvic Clocks . . . . *(page 92)*

Shoulder Drops and Variation . . . . *(page 80)*

Spine Curls with Ribcage Closure . . . . *(page 82)*

Hip Rolls . . . . *(page 93)*

Dart . . . . *(page 94)*

Star . . . . *(page 95)*

Table Top (after 6 weeks) . . . . *(page 96)*

Rest Position . . . . *(page 98)*

Side Reach . . . . *(page 100)*

Roll Downs . . . . *(page 102)*

Pelvic Floor Control . . . . *(page 104)*

From the Early Pregnancy Programme

Knee Rolls . . . . *(page 116)*

Nose Spirals . . . . *(page 117)*

Pelvic Stability Variation . . . . *(page 118)*

Knee Circles . . . . *(page 120)*

Star Variation . . . . *(page 123)*

Cat (after 6 weeks, leave Oblique Cat until you feel

   back to normal) . . . . *(page 124)*

Seated Waist Twist . . . . *(page 126)*

Tennis Ball Rising . . . . *(page 127)*

Foot exercises . . . . *(page 128–131)*

From the Later Pregnancy Programme

Hip Hinge . . . . *(page 152)*

Pilates Squat . . . . *(page 153)*

Dumb Waiter and Variation . . . . *(page 157)*

Chest Expansion . . . . *(page 154)*

Chest Expansion plus Rotation . . . . *(page 155)*

Seated Scapular Squeeze . . . . *(page 158)*

Wrist Circles . . . . *(page 159)*

Arm Openings . . . . *(page 160)*

Oyster . . . . *(page 161)*

Side-lying Circles . . . . *(page 166)*

Seated Zig Zags . . . . *(page 164)*

Calf Stretch . . . . *(page 163)*

The Flower . . . . *(page 167)*

Pelvic Rocking . . . . *(page 180)*

Tail Swish . . . . *(page 182)*

The following may be added once your abdominal divide (diastasis recti) is less than 2cm and there is no doming. (If you've had a caesarean section wait for 5 months before adding to your programme):

Curl Ups . . . . *(page 72)*

Curl Ups with Knee Openings . . . . *(page 84)*

Curl Ups with Leg Extension . . . . *(page 121)*

Oblique Curls may be added when everything is

   back to normal . . . . *(page 86)*

Now that we have a exercise list, we can put some sample workouts together. As we mentioned before, if you put your own workouts together, try to include some spinal flexion, rotation, extension and side flexion. Balance upper and lower body work.

Normal delivery workout

No diastasis recti or special problems. 6 weeks after the birth

Nose Spirals . . . . *(page 117)*

Shoulder Drops . . . . *(page 80)*

Knee Circles . . . . *(page 120)*

Arms Raised Unilateral Band Pull: Single Knee Fold *(page 205)*

Ribcage Closure with Leg Slide . . . . *(page 202)*

Spine Curl with Arm Flies . . . . *(page 200)*

Curl Ups . . . . *(page 72)*

Hip Rolls . . . . *(page 93)*

Oyster . . . . *(page 161)*

Crawling Lizard (small pillow under pelvis if needed)

. . . . *(page 208)*

Star . . . . *(page 95)*

Cat . . . . *(page 124)*

Rest Position . . . . *(page 98)*

Pelvic Floor Control (seated) . . . . *(page 104)*

The Emergency Stop . . . . *(page 106)*

Foot exercises . . . . *(page 128–131)*

Pelvic Floor: Pilates Wide-leg Stance . . . . . . *(page 211)*

Dumb Waiter (standing) . . . . *(page 157)*

Standing Side Reach . . . . *(page 100)*

Roll Downs (against the wall) . . . . *(page 102)*

Caesarean Section workout

After medical clearance:

Neck Rolls . . . . *(page 54)*

Pelvic Tilts . . . . *(page 197)*

Ribcage Closure . . . . *(page 68)*

Single Knee Folds . . . . *(page 63)*

Arms Raised Unilateral Band Pull: Leg Slides . . . *(page 205)*

Spine Curls with Support . . . . *(page 199)*

Creeping Toes (up the wall) . . . . *(page 130)*

Dart (small pillow under pelvis if needed) . . . . . *(page 94)*

Diamond Press (small pillow under pelvis

if needed) . . . . *(page 122)*

Cat . . . . *(page 124)*

Rest Position . . . . *(page 198)*

Arm Openings . . . . *(page 160)*

Side Reach (seated on a chair) do not stretch

too far) . . . . *(page 100)*

Pelvic Floor Control exercises . . . . *(page 104–109)*

Chest Expansion . . . . *(page 154)*

Pelvic Floor: Standing . . . . *(page 211)*

Tennis Ball Rising . . . . *(page 127)*

Scarf Breathing . . . . *(pages 56–57)*

Diastasis Recti workout

Nose Spirals . . . . *(page 117)*

Pelvic Tilts . . . . *(page 197)*

Ribcage Closure . . . . *(page 68)*

Arms Raised Unilateral Band Pull: Single Knee Fold

. . . . *(page 205)*

Arms Raised Bilateral Band Pull: Leg Slide . . . . *(page 204)*

Arms Raised Unilateral Band Pull: Knee Opening *(page 205)*

Spine Curls with Arm Flies . . . . *(page 200)*

Assisted Curl Ups . . . . *(page 206)*

Knee Rolls . . . . *(page 116)*

Cobra Prep (small pillow under pelvis if needed) *(page 207)*

Table Top (keep contact with mat) . . . . *(page 96)*

Rest Position . . . . *(page 98)*

Oyster . . . . *(page 161)*

Pelvic Floor Control (seated) . . . . *(page 104)*

Mexican Wave . . . . *(page 129)*

Waist Twist (standing) . . . . *(page 126)*

Standing Side Reach (caution do not over reach) *(page 100)*

Pilates Squat . . . . *(page 153)*

Working Out with Your Baby

As wonderful as it is being a new mother, there will be times when you are going to need some peace and quiet. Try to take a few moments each day to practise your Pilates alone, where you can focus on yourself and how you are feeling. Motherhood can be very tiring. Try to take note of how your body feels.

If you feel stressed, try the Tension Release exercise. Or just sit quietly and breathe…

But let's be honest, in these early weeks and months you may find you have very little 'me' time. Yet these early weeks are crucial for mending your abdominals and preventing any long-term joint problems. You are still going to need to do your exercises. The solution lies in getting your baby involved in your workout. The added bonus is that you can, at the same time, help your baby's development.

Whenever your baby is asleep, the safest position is lying on their back. But if they spend all their time on their back, the head can flatten a bit. This is not usually serious and will probably correct itself within a year, but it can be avoided. This is just one of the reasons why, when baby is awake, we want to let them play in as many different positions as possible. This will also stimulate them and help encourage their movement skills and development (yes, we catch our future clients young!).

For the first few months your baby will be unable to sit up unaided. They will need support. While every baby will develop at their own rate, most babies' development starts to speed up from about 6 weeks on. At about 8 weeks you will notice that they grasp and shake the toys you give them. If the toy makes a noise, baby's eyes follow the noise. This early grasping is important for their hand to eye co-ordination. By 12 weeks they've perfected this and are looking for more things to grab. Glasses, if you wear them, seem to be popular!

In the early weeks you will have supported their head for them, but by 12 weeks, they will have more control of their head. The only time you will need to support it is if you pick them up or move them quickly and they haven't time to react.

Now you can help develop your baby's head control in a variety of ways. For example, when lying in their cot your baby may prefer to turn their head one way to look at a favourite mobile. Alternate which side you place the mobile as it's important that they learn to turn their head both ways. In the same way, when you are exercising, if your baby is on their back and has woken up, position your baby on alternate sides of the mat so that they have to turn their head different ways to look at you.

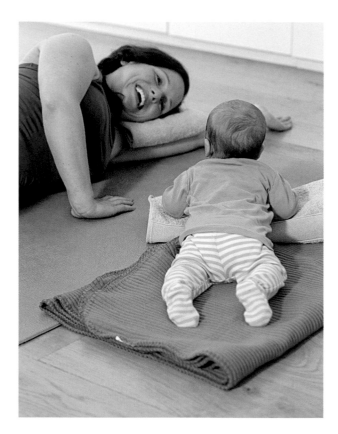

Whenever it is possible, when your baby is awake, place them on their front. Never allow them to fall asleep on their front, you must supervise them.

The general guideline is: **Back to Sleep, Front to Play**

By placing your baby on their front you will be encouraging them to lift their head, helping to develop their spinal curves. By 3 months they will be lifting their chin up. You can help encourage them by placing a rolled up towel under their chest and arms.

This will give them a bit more support. They will not be able to stay there for long. But by about 4 months they should be able to hold their head clear of the floor when they are laid on their front. By being on their front at different angles to your mat you will encourage this head control as they lift their head to look at you.

As they grow, lying on their front also encourages them to start crawling, especially if you place their toys or your mat just out of reach! Some babies start crawling at 6 months, others not until 10 months. Some seem content to move around by shuffling on their bottoms!

With a bit of forethought, when you are exercising, you can also plan to include your baby in such a way as you can continue to bond with them but also help their motor skills. Then not only will you be working on your muscle strength and co-ordination, your baby will too!

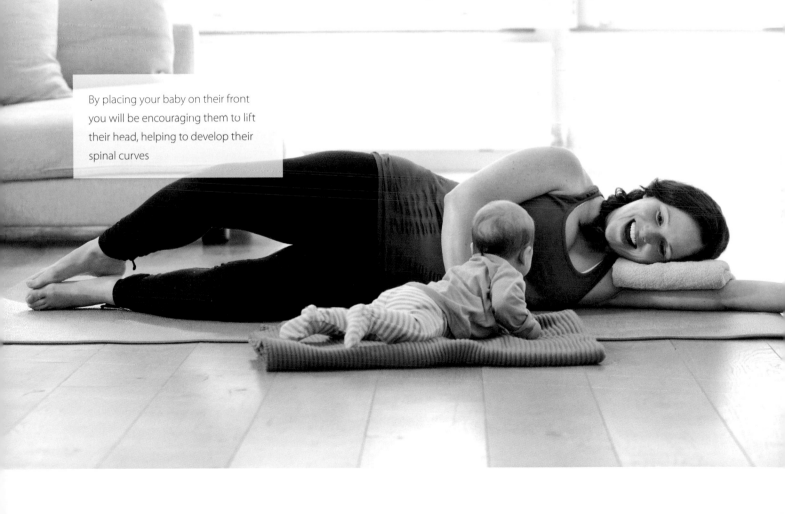

By placing your baby on their front you will be encouraging them to lift their head, helping to develop their spinal curves

Baby Workout Positions

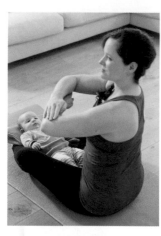
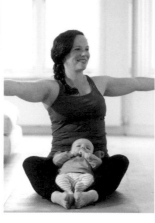
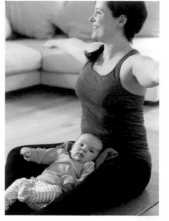

By varying baby's position you can stimulate them. In addition to the position on the previous page try the following.

Your baby will enjoy the session more if they can see you.

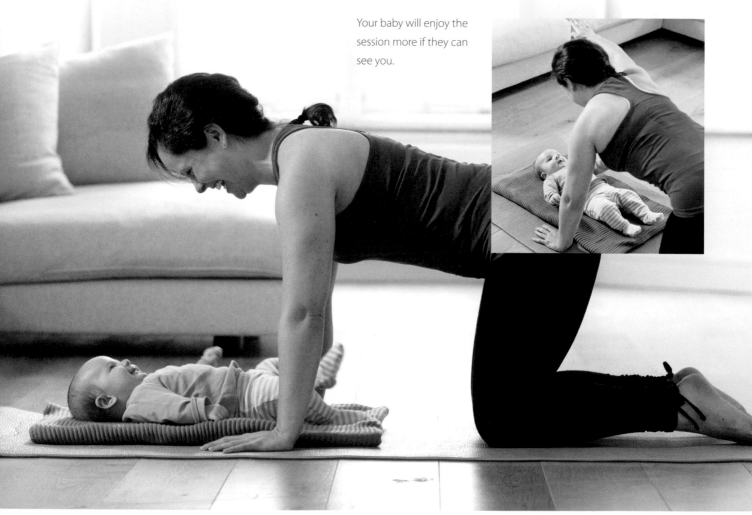

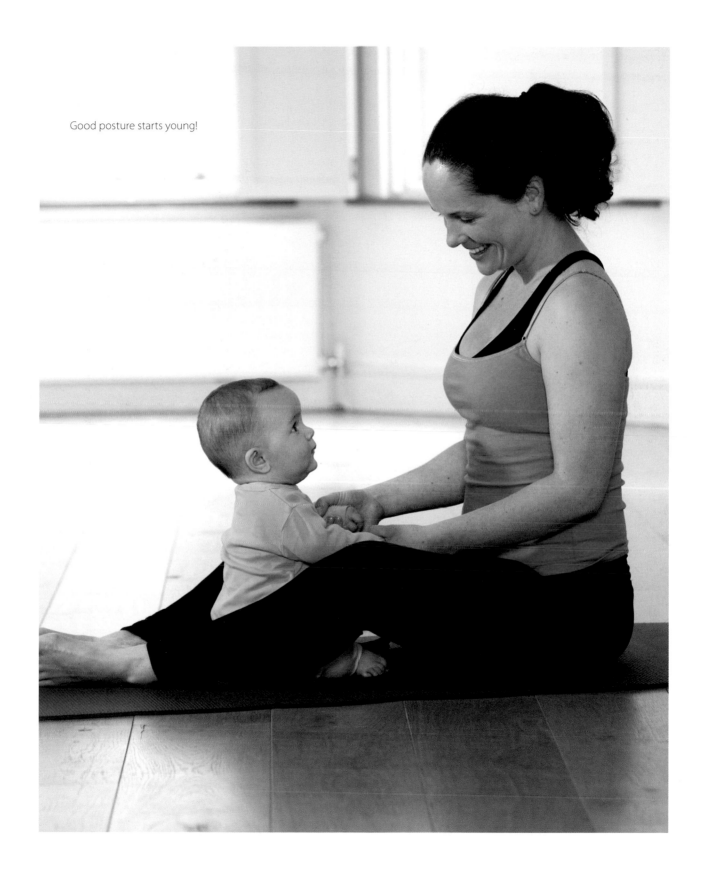

Good posture starts young!

Tips for Good Posture when Caring for Your Baby

Most of your baby-caring activities involve forward bending, and you may find that you have to sit a lot as you feed and play with the baby. You also have to carry your baby around with you. So here are some useful tips on how to protect your back as you look after your new child.

Lifting *Refresh your memory of good lifting techniques on page 145.*

Carrying baby Babies never like to be far from their mothers and most like to be carried around for several hours daily. This can be challenging to a busy new mum. There are some wonderful baby carriers available that are designed to reduce the strain on your back. Generally mothers report that the sling carriers create less strain and appear more comfortable for the baby.

When you are holding baby, hold them close to your body. As they get older try to avoid carrying them on one hip, as it loads the spine and pelvis asymmetrically. Or if you must, at least alternate hips on a regular basis!

Feeding Whether you are breastfeeding or bottle-feeding, try to sit in a comfortable but upright chair with your back supported; if necessary use extra cushions

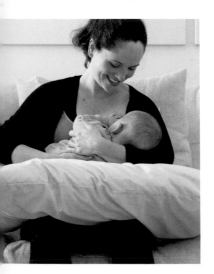

and pillows to ensure that you do not slump down and put pressure on your spine.

Place a pillow on your lap so that the baby is supported too. It might take some time to find the right position. If you are breastfeeding and your baby wants to feed from your left breast, you can cradle your baby in your right arm (which in turn can be supported by the pillow).

Hold your baby so that their body is in a straight line, their stomach to your stomach. In this way their head and neck are not twisted. If you are bottle-feeding, try feeding from both sides. It will give your arms and shoulders a break and is a more natural way to feed.

Nappy changing Changing stations and changing mats that fit across the cot are a must to avoid constantly lying baby on the floor, bending over and lifting baby back up again. Kneeling at the side of a bed is also a better option, but you may need a knee support to help avoid strain.

Prams and buggies The handle height on the buggy or pram may not have been the first consideration when you bought it from the shop, but may be a problem three months in! Handle extensions are available from baby accessory stores and can make a considerable difference to your posture. There are some great pushchairs and buggies on the market which have extendable handles. These are ideal if you or your partner are tall as it helps you to avoid tipping forward at the hips or shoulders when pushing pram, especially on an uphill climb.

Car seats Avoid lifting your baby while they are still in the car seat, out or into the car. This difficult manoeuvre involves bending and twisting and lifting simultaneously – all at a time when your back is still vulnerable.

General exercise Pilates exercises are a safe way to prepare a new mum's body for return to other forms of exercise. But we are not a cardiovascular activity. While you should not do excessive cardiovascular workouts (these may compromise your milk supply if you are breastfeeding) you do need to keep your heart healthy. Symmetrical activities such as brisk walking, swimming, gentle jogging are fine but avoid asymmetrical activities such as tennis, golf, squash until you feel back to normal.

Cardiovascular Activities during Pregnancy and the Postnatal Period

If you did aerobic-type exercise before you became pregnant, with medical permission, you should be able to continue to do some aerobic activities through your pregnancy.

Choose your activities carefully. Remember that your baby is at risk from trauma. We have seen how your spatial awareness is affected by your hormones, how your centre of gravity has shifted. Together this means that you are more at risk of falling.

Exercises to avoid

Scuba diving, high altitude activities, activities with high risk of falls, activities with a high risk of abdominal trauma.

General exercise guidelines

* Exercise should be regular – 30 minutes five times a week, but a day's exercise can be cumulative, for example 3 x 10 minutes brisk walking.

* For pregnancy, exercise should be at an intensity sufficient to increase heart rate up to 70 per cent of maximum (estimated maximum is 220 less age). *Note:* As blood volume increases during pregnancy, the heart will have to work harder. As a general guideline, maternal pulse rate should not exceed 150 beats per minute.

* Wear a supportive, non-wired bra.

* Do not allow your temperature to exceed 38°C. Strenuous exercise may cause increased core body temperature and your baby is not able to lose heat and perspire as you do. For the same reason never exercise with a temperature. Avoid the heat of the day. If indoors, use a well-ventilated cool room. Avoid also saunas/jacuzzis and hot tubs.

* Avoid polluted traffic areas. If walking/running in streets, let someone know where you are going and the time when you are due back.

* Keep hydrated.

* If you experience heavy urine leakage or pelvic pressure seek medical advice.

* When exercising, the glucose levels available to the baby may be decreased and may result in a lower weight of the baby – so, avoid allowing your blood sugar levels to drop. Keep them stable by eating high quality carbohydrates 2–3 hours before exercise.

* Postnatal: be aware that any strenuous type of exercise may drain your energy levels. Exercise burns calories so if you are breastfeeding and doing aerobic activities you must make sure to increase your food and water intake accordingly.

* If you have any back or pelvic problems, avoid asymmetrical activities such as tennis, golf, squash until you feel back to normal.

Above all, for pregnancy and the postnatal period, any activity should make you feel good not exhausted.

Index

A

abdominal divide 193–195
Abdominal Hollowing 60
abdominal muscles 134–135
    girdle 23–241
air embolism 148
alignment 32
    postnatal 196
Ankle Circles 131
antenatal programme, using 11
arches, working 128
Arm Flies 200
Arm Openings 160
Arms Raised 203
    bilateral band pulls, with 204
    unilateral band pulls 205
Assisted Curl Ups 206

B

baby, working out with 213–217
birth
    anterior presentation 179
    breech 179
    caesarean 191–192
    changing body after 188–189
    posterior presentation 179
    preparing for 170–185
    transverse 179
blood pressure 15–16
Body Mass Index 76–77
Braxton Hicks contractions 139
breasts, increase in 137
breathing
    deep abdominal 108
    exhalation 15
    general anaesthetic, exercise
        after 192
    inhalation 15
    late pregnancy, in 139
    mechanism 14–15
    pelvic floor, and 107–108
    postnatal 196
    posture, and 56

pregnancy hormones, effect of 15
    purpose of 14
    Scarf 56–57
    second stage of labour, in 185
    types of 56

C

caesarean birth 191–192
    workout 212
Calf Stretch 163
cardiovascular activities 219
carpal tunnnel syndrome 140–141
Cat, The 124–125
    Oblique Cat 125
centre, finding 60
centring 58–59
    postnatal 196
Cervical Nod 55
cervix 13
    effacement and dilation 171
chair, getting up from 144
Chest Expansion 154
    plus rotation 155
Chest Extension 156
Chin Tucks 54–55
circulation exercises 192
Cobra Prep 207
Compass 42–43
    wall slide position, in 43
core connection 60
core muscles, engaging 59
core stability 59
Crawling Lizard 208–209
Creeping Toes 130
Curl Ups 72
    Assisted 206
    Knee Openings, with 84–85
    Leg Extensions, with 121
    Oblique 86–87
    Oblique with Opposite Leg Slide 87

D

Dart 94
desk, posture at 142–143
Diamond Press 122

Diastasis Recti 24, 194–195
    workout 212
dilation of cervix 171
Dimmer Switch 59
Double Knee Folds 64–65
Dumb Waiter 157

E

Emergency Stop 106
exercise
    birth, after, medical permission for 189
    caesarean birth, after 192
    contraindications 28–29
    doctor, consulting 78
    early pregnancy, in 114
    late pregnancy, guidelines for 148
    postnatal 218–219
    safety 28
    stopping 29
exercise starting positions
    compass 42–43
    Four-point Kneeling 46–47
    High Kneeling 48
    Pilates stance 52
    prone 49
    relaxation position 40–41
    seated 44–45
    side-lying 50–51
episiotomy 172

F

fallopian tubes 13
feet
    arches, working 128
    Creeping Toes 130
    foot exercises 128–131
    heel pain 141
    Mexican Wave 129
fimbria 13
Floating Arms 66–67
floor, getting onto 146–147
Flower, the 167
Four-point Kneeling 61
Four-point Kneeling Positions
    46–47, 180

Free-standing Partner Squats 175
fundus 12

G

getting onto the floor 147
getting up from a chair 144
girdle of strength 23–25

H

haemo-dilation 16
headaches 29
heel pain 141
high kneeling position 48
Hip Hinge 152
Hip Rolls 93

I

'In Between Breath' Zip 61

K

Knee Circles 203, 120
    arms raised with bilateral band
        pulls 204
    arms raised with unilateral band
        pulls 205
Knee Folds
    Double 64–65
    Single 63, 203–205
Knee Openings 63, 203
    arms raised with bilateral band
        pulls 204
    arms raised with unilateral band
        pulls 205
    Curl Ups, with 84–85
    Spine Curls with 201
Knee Rolls 116–117

L

labour
    exercises 172
    first stage 170–183
    Free-standing Partner Squats 175
    managing 170
    Partner Squatting 174
    phases of 170

preparing for 170–185
relaxation during 176–177
relaxation position 177
second stage 184–185
tension release exercises 178
third stage 185
transitions 184–185

late pregnancy
    breasts, increase in 137
    breathing 139
    chair, getting up from 144
    clothing and footwear 148
    common conditions 138–139
    desk, posture at 142–143
    digestion in 135
    exercise guidelines 148
    floor, getting onto 146–147
    joints 138
    lifting and carrying well 145
    Pilates fundamentals for 149–150
    programme for 134–167
    sleeping 145
    workouts 151
Leg Slides 58, 62, 203
    arms raised with bilateral band
        pulls 204
    arms raised with unilateral band
        pulls 205
    Oblique Curl Ups, with 87
    Ribcage Closure, with 202
lifting and carrying well 145
ligamentous laxity 17-18
Long Frog 44
lungs 14

M

maternal organs 12
Mexican Wave 129
miscarriage, risk of 29
mobility 58–59, 71
mood changes after birth 190–191
Neck Rolls 54

N

Nose Spirals 117

O

Oblique Cat 125
Oblique Curl Ups 86–87
    Opposite Leg Slide, with 87
Oblique Rest position 125
oedema 16
ovaries 13
overweight 77
Oyster 161

P

Partner Squatting 174
    Free-standing Partner Squats 175
pelvic bones 17
pelvic canal 17
Pelvic Clocks 92
Pelvic Elevator 105
pelvic floor
    birth, after 190
    breathing, and 107–108
    control 104
    engaged 25
    exercises 104–109
    facts 104
    muscles 24
    release 140
    rest, at 25
    trampoline 25
pelvic girdle pain 193
pelvic laxity 17–18
pelvic organs 12
Pelvic Rocking 180–181
pelvic stability exercises 198
Pelvic Stability Variations 118–119
Pelvic Tilts 197
Pilates
    after birth 188–219
    antenatal 9, 11
    antenatal programme, using 11
    benefits of 9
    equipment 28
    fundamentals 32–33
    late pregnancy, fundamentals for
        149–150
    postnatal 9

e-pregnancy 9
  safety 28
  tension, release of 26
Pilates Squat 153
Pilates Stance 52, 211
Pilates Wide Leg Stance 211
Pillow Squeeze 106–106
placenta 13
postnatal pelvic stability exercises
    203–205
postnatal programme 196
postnatal workouts 212–212
posture
  assessing 34–35
  check 137
  daily activities, in 142
  pregnancy, in 19–22
  while caring for baby 218–219
pregnancy
  abdominal muscles 134–135
  blood volume, increase in 15
  breathing 14–15
  changing body, 0-16 weeks 112–113
  changing body, 16 weeks-full term
    134
  early, programme for 112–131
  exercise guidelines, first weeks
    114
  gastrointestinal system, effect on
    16
  heart rate, increase in 15
  hormonal influences 14–16
  later, programme for 134–167 *see
    also late pregnancy*
  lymphatic fluid, increase in 16
  oedema 16
  pins and needles during 140–141
  posture, changes in 19–22
  preparing for 76–107
  trimesters 12
  urine flow, increase in 16
  uterine vascular system, blood
    volume in 16
  weight gain in 113–114
prone positions 49

R
Rec Check 195
relaxation 26
relaxation position 40–41
Rest Position 98–99
Ribcage Closure 68–69
  Spine Curls, with 82–83
  Wall Slide, in 69
ribcage changes 189
Ribcage Closure and Leg Slides 202
Roll Downs 102–103

S
sacrospinous ligament 18
sacrotuberous ligament 18
Scarf Breathing 56–57
Seated Scapular Squeeze 158
seated starting positions
    chair, on 45
    Long Frog 44
    mat, on 44
    wall 44
Seated Waist Twist 126
Seated Zig Zags 164–165
Security Barrier 67
Shhhh, the 189
Shoulder Drops 80
    variation 1 81
    variation 2 81
Side Reach 100–101
Side-lying Circles 166
side-lying positions 50–51
Single Knee Folds 63, 203
    arms raised with bilateral band
      pulls 204
    arms raised with unilateral band
      pulls 205
Single Leg Stretch 71
    Stage 1 88–89
    Stage 2 90–91
sleeping in pregnancy 145
Spine Curls 58, 72
    Arm Flies, with 200
    Knee Openings, with 201
    Ribcage Closure, with 82–83

Spine Curls with Support 199
spine, natural curves of 33
stability 58–59
Standing Alignment 53
standing pelvic floor exercises
    210–211
Star 95
Star Variation 123
Starfish 70
stress incontinence 106
stretching 71
Supine Hypotension Syndrome 136
symphysis pubis dysfunction 18, 193

T
Table Top
    Stage 1 96
    Stage 2 97
Tail Swish 182–183
Tennis Ball Rising 127
tension release exercises 178

U
umbilical cord 13
underweight 77
uterus 12–13

V
vagina 13
    air embolism 148

W
Walking on the Spot 161
Wall Slides 210
    Compass 43
    Ribcage Closure 69
    variation A 36–37
    variation B 38–39
Wind Zip 60
Working the Arches 128
Wrist Circles 159
Wrist Stretches 181

Further Information

Body Control Pilates

Body Control Pilates was founded in 1995 with a vision to make the benefits of Pilates as accessible as possible to the average person, irrespective of age, income and fitness level. Our unique programme takes you progressively and safely towards the Joseph Pilates's original work. We have always believed that it is the quality of teaching which defines good Pilates and are proud that Body Control Pilates is now widely seen as a benchmark for safe and effective mat and machine teaching of the highest quality.

Body Control Pilates' HQ is in Bloomsbury in the heart of London, where we operate studios, public classes, teacher training and development courses. We also have training partners throughout the world in countries such as China, South Africa, South Korea, Canada, Denmark, Norway, Portugal and Lithuania.

A list of all certified Body Control Pilates teachers can be found at our websites www.bodycontrol.co.uk and www.bodycontrolpilates.com

UK

Chartered Society of Physiotherapists
www.csp.org.uk

Chartered Physiotherapists in Women's Health
www.acpwh.org.uk

General Chiropractic Council
www.gcc-uk.org

General Osteopathic Council
www.osteopathy.org.uk

National Health Service
www.nhs.uk

Postnatal depression (NHS)
http://www.nhs.uk/Conditions/Postnataldepression/Pages/Diagnosis.aspx

The Association for Postnatal Illness
www.apni.org

Royal College of Obstetricians and Gynaecologists
http://www.rcog.org.uk

Royal College of Midwives
www.rcm.org.uk

Independent Midwives
www.independentmidwives.org.uk

National Childbirth Trust (NCT)
http://www.nct.org.uk

Hypnobirthing
www.thehypnobirthingcentre.co.uk

Doulas
www.doula.org.uk

Pelvic girdle pain charity support group
www.pelvicpartnership.org.uk

Carpal tunnel wrist splints
www.physioroom.com

Serola belt and maternity belt
www.physiotherapystore.com/Maternity

Healthy Eating During Pregnancy
Erika Lenkert with Brooke Alpert MS RD CDN, Kyle Books

What to Expect When You're Expecting, Heidi E Murkoff and Sharon Mazel, Simon & Schuster

IRELAND

Irish Childbirth Trust
www.cuidiu-ict.ie

Irish Nurses and Midwives Organisation
www.inmo.ie

Maeve Whelan physiotherapy
www.pelvicphysiotherapy.com

USA AND CANADA

The American Chiropractic Association
www.acatoday.org

American Osteopathic Association
www.osteopathic.org

American College of Nurse-Midwives
www.midwife.org

Childbirth and Postpartum Professional Association of Canada
www.cappacanada.ca

AUSTRALIA

Australian College of Midwives
www.midwivesaustralia.com

Childbirth Australia
www.childbirth.org.au

NEW ZEALAND

The New Zealand College of Midwives
www.midwife.org.nz

SOUTH AFRICA

Childbirth Educators / Midwives
www.pregnant2day.co.za

Acknowledgements

Where do I start? I have been constantly blown away by the kindness and generosity of everyone who has worked on this book and everyone who has supported Leigh and I over the last 15 years as we have built Body Control Pilates.

Our medical consultant for the book, Kate, managed to make the whole experience of writing this great fun. I was so lucky to have her on board as she shared her medical knowledge and also her personal experience as mother to the gorgeous Will and Grace!

Heartfelt thanks also to Gail Hillier, Body Control Pilates teacher and midwife who proofread the book and whose insightful comments kept me on track and up to date with current midwifery advice.

Ruth, thank you so much for your kind words in the foreword and for all the support you have given to Body Control Pilates.

Thanks too to the lovely Linda who so kindly read through the manuscript and who has so brightened up my Tuesday mornings!

Then there's Jennifer, our editor, whose patience was limitless and who has kept a sure and steady hand at the helm from the book's conception through to print. She even became pregnant during the process – now there's dedication to duty!
Big Dan, Young Dan, many thanks for making the photoshoot so relaxed, your skills have made this book a work of art! Jane, our designer, how you fitted it all I'll never know, it looks just stunning. Marie, your make-up worked its usual magic – thank you!

Words are not enough to express my thanks to the stunning models who battled across London on some of the hottest days of the year. They all look amazing: Preparing for Pregnancy and Fundamentals models: Claire, Kate, Anaya and Sally. Early Pregnancy models: Eilis and Lina. (A confession here and an apology. The more observant amongst you may well notice that Lina was further on in her pregnancy than 16 weeks at the time of the shoot. The photography dates kept moving back and her gorgeous bump kept growing. I hope you will all forgive us this small transgression!). Later Pregnancy models: Lindsay, Stephanie, Elena, Sally and Joy. Postnatal models: Sarah Warden and the handsome Matteo, who won all our hearts!

I am very fortunate to count as clients some of the most stunning women from the world of TV and movies, but I can honestly say that, Sophie, they don't come any kinder, more beautiful or more genuine than you. Thank you so much for the cover quote. We all adore you and your fabulous family!

And last, but by no means least, I would like to dedicate this book to my beautiful daughters Rebecca and Emily and to my dear mother Doris Ada Baker, who gave me the best possible start in life and whom I miss daily.